D1563792

"You Bring Out the Music in Me": Music in Nursing Homes

"You Bring Out the Music in Me": Music in Nursing Homes

Beckie Karras
Editor

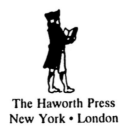

The Haworth Press
New York • London

"You Bring Out the Music in Me": Music in Nursing Homes has also been published as *Activities, Adaptation & Aging*, Volume 10, Numbers 1/2 1987.

The Haworth Press, Inc. 10 Alice Street, Binghamton, NY 13904-1580
EUROSPAN/Haworth, 3 Henrietta Street, London WC2E 8LU England

Library of Congress Cataloging-In-Publication Data

"You bring out the music in me" Beckie Karras, editor.
    p. cm.
    "Has also been published as Activities, adaptation & aging, v. 10, numbers 1/2, 1987" — T.p. verso
    Includes bibliographies.
    ISBN 0-86656-699-6
    1. Music therapy for the aged. 2. Nursing homes — Recreational activities. I. Karras, Beckie.
ML3920.Y68 1987
615.8'5154 — dc19

                                           87-22931
                                              CIP
                                              MN

"You Bring Out the Music in Me": Music in Nursing Homes

CONTENTS

ETCHINGS

Music as Sleep Therapy   123
Vida Hickerson

Resource List   125
Compiled by Michael Lewallen

Introduction

Mr. K. is an 86-year-old immigrant from China, now living in a nursing home and vaguely aware of where he is. Having spent most of his life in China, he speaks little English and knows even less about American music. Yet at the weekly sing-alongs, he smiles, claps, dances, and even "directs" the music.

Mrs. B. is in the final stages of Alzheimer's disease and spends her days sing-songing "mamamama." Yet if earphones are put on her, with music playing softly in her head, her eyes brighten, her sing-song stops, and she smiles and sways to the music with the therapist working with her.

Mr. L., confused and disabled from Parkinson's disease, can only stand with support, yet each Friday he comes to Happy Hour and stands with the administrator, singing "I'm in Love With You, Honey."

Mrs. F. suffered both a stroke and a hip fracture and entered the nursing home for a long rehabilitation to restore her mobility and some of her speech. We watched her progress at our weekly dance parties as she "sang" and "danced" in her wheelchair, until finally that magic day came that she was able to stand and then dance the "two-step" away from her chair.

Saying that "music is the universal language" has special meaning among the elderly, because there are *very* few people whom music cannot reach. Regardless of one's language, culture, or abilities, music "speaks" to all of us. It motivates, enriches, touches, relaxes, energizes. From "Rock-a-bye-Baby" to "Blest Be the Tie That Binds," our lives are filled with music.

To paraphrase an old commercial. "A home without music is like a home without sunshine." Bringing more music into nursing homes, and more sunshine, is what this book is about.

The articles encompass both music therapy practice in gerontology as well as practical ideas and suggestions for activities directors who want to use music in their nursing home activities programs. The book begins with a history of music therapy, examines the need for research in the field, moves into discussions of music in groups and music with individuals, and ends with a resource list of music materials.

The group which put together this book, Music Therapists in Gerontology, began as a support group. In May of 1984, Louise Lynch and I met as fellow music therapists to discuss a stroke patient in need of one-to-one music therapy. The meeting was very fruitful and stimulating, as we discovered common concerns and ideas in our practice of music therapy with older people. Two months after this first meeting, we brought together music therapists who were doing similar work in other nursing homes in the Washington, D.C. area. We gave ourselves a name and began meeting every two months.

Initially, we shared ideas and resources, as well as the "trials and tribulations" of our work. After meeting for a little over a year, we wanted to find a focus for the group and began work on a video project, a short film that would give an overview of the many ways music therapy can be used in the nursing home setting. Soon after the filming on this was completed, in the spring of 1986, we enthusiastically began work on this present volume of "Activities, Adaptation and Aging."

We wish to express our appreciation to Phyllis Foster, editor of the "Activities, Adaptation, and Aging" journal, for giving us the opportunity to write about our work and for her support and encouragement during the writing process.

We also want to gratefully acknowledge the work of Loretta Smith, RMT, who provided valuable recommendations on the editing of several of the manuscripts, and to Jack Colligan who did final proofreading.

In closing, since I believe in letting people speak for themselves, I would like to share the poetry of two nursing home residents I have known. Both poems were written while listening to Pachelbel's "Canon in D."

Beckie Karras
Project Coordinator

The music I hear now
Unlocks in me a nice first ball,
Dancing and flirting with a loved one;
It takes me to my old home town
Where I grew up and went to school
And found my husband;
It unlocks in me a dream of
Happiness and enjoyment;
It further takes me to the theater,
Where I watched nice operas being performed;
It makes me feel that I want
To dance and dance —
I could have danced all night!
The music unlocks in me
The secret wish of being able
To sing, marvelling at people
Like Beverly Sills who can
Remember the whole opera.

Anna Goldschmidt

Music is like love —
It takes you to a land of dreams;
Who can compare with that
Beautiful feeling of make believe?

Pauline Immerman

Music Therapy:
Its Historical Relationships
and Value in Programs
for the Long-Term Care Setting

Louise Lynch

SUMMARY. This article deals with the historical relationships of music, medicine and healing and how music can effectively be used in relaxation and art groups with the elderly to encourage expression of feelings and increase socialization.

> "There is a Charm: a Power that sways the breast;
> Bids every Passion revel or be still;
> Inspires with Rage, or all your Cares dissolves;
> Can soothe Distraction, and almost Despair.
> That Power is Music."
>
> *John Armstrong*
> *The Art of Preserving Health (1744)*

The powerful effects of music upon healing have been known since early man, but only today is the relationship between music

---

Louise Lynch, RMT-BC, is a Registered Music Therapist with a Music Therapy degree from Catholic University, Washington, DC. She is working on her Masters in Gerontology/Psychology from Hood College, Frederick, MD. She is currently the Activities Director for the National Lutheran Home in Rockville, MD. She designed and developed a therapeutic program for the special Dementia Unit at the Hebrew Home of Greater Washington. She is a national speaker and workshop leader in working with the Alzheimer patient and in setting up and managing programs for Alzheimer units. She is also a co-founder, with Beckie Karras, of the Washington, DC area Music Therapists in Gerontology.

and medicine being scientifically researched and used therapeutically. Music involves man's mind, body, spirit and emotions closely intertwined with his personality, education, social and cultural environments. Music is built on harmonic relationships just as social harmony is dependent on interpersonal relationships.

The association of music and the magic of healing begins with the fact that music is an integral part of human life through sound. We are not only capable of making sound within ourselves, but we are surrounded by sounds of nature in the environment. We use sound through our vocal chords to communicate with one another so it seems only natural that primitive man might have seen the sounds of nature as communication with invisible spirits.

The tribal musician in primitive times was usually a person with some innate psychic ability, very perceptive but usually remarkably unstable emotionally. He had great importance and power within the tribe and it was thought that he could call upon the spirits by imitating their sounds. His specific function was to find the right song for each particular illness or healing procedure. Even though each tribe had its own intertwined religious and magic philosophy of disease and illness, it was the general belief of all tribes that the sick person was an innocent victim of secret powers of the spirits.

In addition to finding songs appropriate to healing, it was the musician's job to use instruments such as drums and rattles which were thought to drive away illness and evil spirits. Often the family and friends of the sick person would join together as a chorus to reinforce the magic of the music. All of these things prepared the person psychologically to help cure himself.

Music played an important part also in the tribal ceremonies of the American Indian. Harmony between man and nature was of utmost importance in Indian life. Health, strength and long life were considered to be the natural condition and illness was disharmony. Songs were used to communicate with the spirits of nature. Ownership of a song belonged to the person who received it in a dream. However, to make the song more powerful, several people would get together to sing it with the owner's permission. The songs used by the medicine man in the healing ceremonies were thought to come from the spirits in dreams or visions, along with directions for curing a particular illness or disease. Drums and rattles were used as in primitive tribes to frighten away evil spirits. Characteristics of Indian songs even today are: irregularity of rhythm or change of accent in the melody; a slow tempo to quiet the patient; and the same tempo of melody and accompaniment creating a monotonous effect. This probably created a semi-hypnotic state.

It was during the early Greek civilization that music and medicine became more closely intertwined. The God Apollo, believed to promote harmony in life and the universe and beauty through the arts of poetry, dancing, and music, was also the founder of medicine. He represented pure intellect and the purest harmony of body and soul. Music and medicine were considered as one in his divine nature. Apollo is thought to have instructed Aesculapius who became the divine symbol of the preventative and the curative powers of nature. Plato felt so strongly about the importance of music to create harmony in one's daily life that he wrote in his Fourth Book of the Republic, "health of mind and body achieved through music." Meinecke sums up other Greek philosophies:

> . . . music is a medicine of the soul. Music was bestowed on man for the sake of effecting harmonious revolutions of the soul within us whenever its rhythmic motions are disturbed. Thus when the soul has lost its harmony, melody and rhythm assist in restoring it to order and concordance. (Meinecke, 1948)

Aristotle claimed that reaction to harmony and rhythm is an inborn trait in all humans and that the soul and harmony are one. He also "ascribed the beneficial and medicinal effects of music to an emotional catharsis." Music provides an outlet for feelings or moods that cannot be verbally described, feelings so deep within that they seem to have no tangible basis. Research shows that music more often produces feelings of rest, joy, sadness, love, longing and reverence while the destructive emotions of fear, anger and jealousy do not seem to be aroused. (Gilman and Paperte, 1952)

The Renaissance reinforced the Greek view that disease was a temporary disruption of harmony in the body. Music was written to honor the saints who protected many from illness. With the advent of more scientific knowledge in the 17th and 18th centuries, the relationship between music and medicine began to be actively studied. The Baroque "Doctrine of Affections" reflected the realization that our deeply rooted emotions are peculiarly responsive to music. As learned people began to try to answer the questions of how music does act upon the mind and body of man and what are its effects, research has opened the doors to the present study and application of music therapy.

Music therapy is defined by Juliette Alvin as, "the controlled use of music in the treatment, rehabilitation, education and training of children and adults suffering from physical, mental or emotional disorder" (Alvin, 1975). Research indicates that there are both physiological and emotional effects produced by music. Since people are now living longer due to new medical technology, music therapy can help alleviate some of the problems faced by the institutionalized elderly. This will be dealt with in depth further into the article.

An understanding of the physical response to music will assist in illustrating the application of music therapy with the elderly. Psychomotor response to music is a natural impulse. Research by Ira M. Altschuler, "Music Therapy Retrospect and Perspective," *Bulletin of the National Association for Music Therapy*, January, 1953, states that:

> . . . the thalamus, which is the seat of all sensation, emotion, and aesthetic feeling, is not involved in mental illness, and that patients who cannot be reached by verbal messages to the brain, can be aroused by music, by way of the thalamus, which when stimulated, automatically relays the sensations to the brain.

This is seen in the involuntary rhythmic response to music by tapping the foot, swaying movement of the body or nodding the head. This rhythmic stimulation is especially useful in establishing contact with disturbed or confused patients, as it offers a nonverbal means of self-expression and the emotional release of conflict through an acceptable social activity.

In addition to instinctive rhythmic response to music, even

patients who cannot be reached verbally often respond by singing the words to a familiar song. Music seems to release emotional tension through expressive reaction to the music. The most important factors in arousing emotional response to the music are a steady rhythm and medium to slow tempo. Regular rhythm encourages physical movement and is especially good for people with restricted activity such as wheelchair patients. Even though they can move only small areas such as head or fingers, they have an inner feeling of greater freedom and control over their bodies. With both ambulatory and wheelchair people, gentle circular movements of most of the upper body is possible; however, care must be taken with moving the head to prevent neck strain and dizziness. Often these simple exercises lead to spontaneous movement and create a feeling of self-confidence as well as physical well-being. Body movement increases circulation, improves breathing capacity, and anxiety is reduced through relaxation exercises.

Changes in pulse rate and respiration are produced by the intensity of the emotional reaction to music. The rhythm of respiration tends to adapt itself to the rhythm of the music, especially as the rhythm gets slower. Music can: increase metabolism; increase or decrease muscular energy; affect respiration and circulation (heart beat, blood pressure and pulse rates). Tempo changes in the music are the chief cause of respiratory changes and as the music becomes more familiar, the physiological changes become more pronounced.

Since everyone is exposed to sound from birth, certain sounds may reveal part of the unconscious personality through memory and association. Often music and rhythm are an important means of communication when feelings are either consciously or intellectually hidden. The sound of some song from the past may be the key to help the patient release long-forgotten memories and under-the-surface feelings.

The institutionalized elderly often become withdrawn and unsociable because they feel deprived and lonely. Music groups can be insurance against loneliness. With music, one is always in communication with the composer as well as with other members of the group. Music groups can help an individual adjust to reality and provide a nonthreatening environment in which to begin again to socialize. Through music, the elderly can be helped to get in touch with and express feelings that may be difficult to verbalize. One method used is to encourage the group to fully relax and allow themselves to go with and respond to the music and the feelings it produces. In this case it is important to match the music to the mood of the group. For example, depressed people often become further depressed and withdraw from cheerful or joyful music. Slow, sad and familiar music will often allow them to feel whatever grief is inside and to express these sad feelings to others in the group. The group itself serves a special purpose by providing a safe environment in which to discuss the feelings provoked by the music.

IMPLEMENTING A RELAXATION GROUP AND AN ART AND MUSIC GROUP

The relaxation group can provide a method for "getting away" from the physical realities of immobility, pain, poor vision, hearing loss and a variety of other disabilities. Using music designed to create a calm atmosphere (see mood music list at end of article), you will begin to set the stage for the relaxation group. I prefer the group to be seated in a circle, if possible, and to use dim or diffused light. Try to conduct this group in a place where there will be no interruptions and where extraneous noise can be kept out. While people are arriving and becoming settled in the circle, I usually use music that is orderly in its harmonic makeup and regular in rhythm. Music of Bach, Vivaldi, Pachelbel or other Baroque composers fits quite nicely here. As the group settles into a regular rhythm, begin to lower the pitch of your voice and slow down your speech until you are verbally guiding the group in a voice pattern that is relatively free of fluctuation. Instruct the group to concentrate on their body rhythm as they breathe in and out. Select one group member who is into a regular pattern and use that person as your focus. Suggest that they may want to close their eyes.

At this point you may continue with the music already established or change to a piece especially chosen to promote imagery and relaxation. Guide the group by gently suggesting that they imagine themselves to be in a place that is especially beautiful for them. It may be a place that they see only in their mind's eye, but it must be free of unpleasantness. Suggest that they imagine themselves free of pain and disabilities. Continue to remind them to concentrate on their body rhythm as they breathe in and out. To relax all body parts, begin either at the head or the feet and work from top to bottom or bottom to top. In an ongoing group you may want to alternate from time to time. To illustrate the routine we will begin at the bottom. Suggest that they begin by concentrating on their feet, moving the toes, being aware of the bones and muscles and how they feel. Ask them to tense the muscles in their feet, hold them tensed for 10 to 20 seconds, and then to let go and relax. Continue to remind them to be aware of their body rhythm as they breathe in and out. Move up to the ankles and calves of the legs, repeat the tensing, relaxation and reminders of body rhythm. Move to the knees and thighs, buttocks, abdomen, ribs, chest, hands (making fists, letting go), arms, shoulders, neck, mouth and jaws, nose and eyes, ending with forehead and scalp. The pattern of tensing and relaxation continues throughout all body parts.

Suggest now that they are feeling very relaxed, warm, and heavy, and that they continue to enjoy their pleasant surroundings. Without talking now, listen to the music for 5-20 minutes, depending on the mood of the group and the session time left. At the end of the allotted time, suggest that they begin to bring to a close the image of their special place and bring themselves back to the room. At the end of each relaxation session have closure by having the group stretch arms, legs and taking several deep breaths. You may want to make verbal closure by asking if the group would like to share their imagery, thoughts and/or feelings.

Many people do not feel comfortable in this kind of relaxation situation at first. It may take several sessions before all the group members are able to allow themselves to fully relax.

When working with the more impaired residents you may find it helpful to simplify your verbal instructions and perhaps to show by example what you want them to do.

This kind of relaxation session is very helpful to staff as well. You may be able to encourage staff to attend a short 10-15 minute session during lunch hour or break.

It is important to remember that music should never be played continuously as background music. There should always be periods of silence between any activity involving music. Don't forget that silence is therapeutic also! Too much sound becomes sensory overload and may increase agitation. The relaxation session helps most residents feel more comfortable, less stressed and generally increases a feeling of well-being.

Art and music groups are another method for providing a non-verbal means of expressing feelings provoked by music.

Choose music designed to elicit specific feelings. (See mood music list at end of article.) Have art materials easily accessible. For this activity you will need to use tables. This is an excellent opportunity for residents to be able to make choices of colors and medium. Pastels, crayons (both regular and oversize non-roll) and poster paint and brushes are good choices. You may need to adapt the brushes by gluing strips of foam rubber around the handle to give more support. To prevent the drawing paper from slipping, secure it to the tabletop with masking tape.

Instruct the group to first listen to the music, being aware of the images that come to mind. Then as the music is played again, ask them to draw whatever feelings are provoked by the music. For the more impaired residents, you may need to make suggestions or to ask them only to choose a color that represents their feeling about the music.

After the project is completed, each person may share his/her picture and feelings about the music with the group.

This activity may be a slow starter as well, since many people do not feel comfortable with materials. You will hear "I can't draw," "This is for children," or other excuses. If you persevere and participate in the activity yourself, you will find most excuses disappear rapidly.

Both the relaxation and art groups are valuable in any activity programming. They provide an opportunity for creative expression of feelings and socialization. Listening to music in these groups often improves general listening skills which can then be transferred to verbal communication and leads to more satisfying social interaction.

In conclusion, there is certainly enough evidence, historically and scientifically, to show that the use of music in therapeutic programs is beneficial. For the elderly, music can play an important role in helping the individual to grow old with greater self-esteem and less loneliness. The ultimate goal of the music therapist in this setting is to help the geriatric patient return to a socially satisfying life.

MOOD MUSIC

Category A. (Happy, Gay, Joyous, Stimulating, Triumphant)

1. Stars and Stripes Forever March — Sousa.
2. William Tell Overture (Finale) — Rossini.
3. Washington Post March — Sousa.
4. Symphony No. 7 in A Major (3rd Movement) — Beethoven.
5. Humoresque — Dvorak.
6. Turkey in the Straw — Folk Song.
7. The Messiah: Hallelujah Chorus — Handel.
8. Ritual Fire Dance (From "El Amor Brujo") — DeFalla.
9. An American in Paris — Gershwin.
10. Mefisto Waltz — Liszt
11. Blue Danube Waltz — Strauss.
12. Die Walkure: Ride of the Valkyries — Wagner.
13. Aida: Grand March — Verdi.
14. Symphony No. 8 — Dvorak.

Category B. (Agitated, Restless, Irritating)

1. Symphonie Fantastique (Finale) — Berlioz.
2. Flight of the Bumblebee — Rimsky-Korsakoff.
3. Sonata, Opus 35, for Piano (lst Movement) — Chopin.
4. Rated-X — Miles Davis.

Category C. (Nostalgic, Sentimental, Soothing, Meditative, Relaxing)

1. Rhapsody in Blue — Gershwin.
2. Liebestraum No. 3 — Liszt.
3. Clair de Lune — Debussy.
4. Lullaby — Brahms.
5. Moonlight Sonata (lst Movement) — Beethoven.

6. Air on the G String — Bach.
7. Waltz of the Flowers (Nutcracker Suite) — Tchaikovsky.
8. Score from "The Lost Weekend" — Rozsa.
9. The Koln Concert — Keith Jarrett.
10. Eastern Peace — Steve Halpern.
11. Renaissance de la Harpe Celtique — Alan Stivall.
12. Ancient Beauty — Do'A.
13. Lullaby from the Womb — Dr. Murooka.
14. Pachelbel Kanon — Munchinger Orchestra.
15. Master of the Bamboo Flute — Sachdev.
16. Serenade to Music (Instrumental Version) — Vaughan Williams.
17. Fantasia on a Theme of Thomas Tallis — Vaughan Williams.
18. A Shrop Shire Lad and On the Banks of Green Willow — George Butterworth.
19. Golden Voyage Series — Ron Dexter.
20. Song of the Seashore — James Galway.
21. Timeless Motion — Daniel Kobialka.
22. Solitudes Series — Environmental Sounds.

Category D. (Prayerful, Reverent)

1. Organ Choral No. 1 — Franck.
2. Mass in B Minor (Crucifixus) — Bach.
3. Xerxes: Largo — Handel.
4. Jesu, Joy of Man's Desiring — Bach.

Category E. (Sad, Melancholy, Grieving, Depressing, Lonely)

1. Sonata, Opus 35 (Funeral March) — Chopin.
2. Romeo and Juliet Overture — Tchaikovsky.
3. Symphony No. 6 ("Pathetique"), 4th movement — Tchaikovsky.
4. Tristan and Isolde — Wagner.
5. Vocalise — Rachmaninoff.
6. Isle of the Dead — Rachmaninoff.

Category F. (Eerie, Weird, Grotesque)

1. Firebird Suite, Part 1 — Stravinsky.
2. La Mer (1st Movement) — Debussy.
3. The Rite of Spring (Part 1) — Stravinsky.

REFERENCES

Alvin, Juliette. *Music Therapy*. New York: Basic Books, 1975.

Benson, Herbert. *The Relaxation Response*. New York: William Morrow and Company, Inc., 1975.

Bonny, Helen L., and Savary, Louis M. *Music and Your Mind*. New York: Harper and Row, 1973.

Bright, Ruth. *Practical Planning in Music Therapy for the Aged*. Lynbrook, New York: Musicgraphics, 1981.

Burnside, Irene Mortenson, ed. *Working With the Elderly*. North Scituate, Mass.: Duxbury Press, 1979.

Capurso, Alexander, et al. *Music and Your Emotions*. New York: Liveright Publishing Corp., 1952.

Drury, Nevill. *Music for Inner Space*. Sydney, Australia: Unity Press, 1985.

Farnsworth, Paul R. *Social Psychology of Music*. New York: Dryden Press, 1958.

Gilman, Leonard, and Paperte, Frances. *Music and Your Emotions*. New York: Liveright Publishing Corp., 1952.

Gaston, E. Thayer, ed. *Music in Therapy*. New York: Macmillan Publishing Co., Inc., 1968.

Halpern, Steven, and Savary, Louis. *Sound Health, The Music and Sounds That Make Us Whole*. New York: Harper and Row, 1985.

Katch, Shelly, and Merle-Fishman, Carol. *The Music Within You*. New York: Simon and Schuster, Inc., 1985.

Levine, Stephen. *A Gradual Awakening*. New York: Anchor Press/Doubleday, 1979.

Levine, Stephen. *Who Dies?* New York: Anchor Press/Doubleday, 1982.

Lingerman, Hal A. *The Healing Energies of Music*. Wheaton, Illinois: The Theosophical Publishing House, 1983.

Meinecke, Bruno. *Music and Medicine*. New York: H. Schuman, 1948.

Rosin, Elizabeth. *Dance in Psychotherapy*. New York: Bureau of Publications, Teachers College, Columbia University, 1957.

Schillian, Dorothy, and Schoen, Max, eds. *Music and Medicine*. New York: H. Schuman, 1948.

Schneider, Erwin H., ed. *Music Therapy 1962*. Lawrence, Kansas: Allen Press, 1963.

Wescott, Juanita. *Magic and Music*. Tucson, Arizona: Abbetira Publications, 1982.

A Justification of Music Therapy in the Nursing Home Setting

Anne W. Lipe

SUMMARY. Many articles which have attempted to justify the use of music or other creative arts therapies with the elderly have done so by stressing the therapeutic benefits inherent within the art form itself. In order for these therapies to survive as a viable treatment medium in the nursing home, the effects of these therapies must be subjected to scientific research methods. The very nature of art forms as therapy makes this task difficult but not insurmountable. It is important to identify which aspects of the activities program can be classified as diversional and which can be classified as therapeutic. Activities professionals need to communicate their observations with other health care disciplines in a systematic, verifiable manner.

There have been numerous articles written in the past fifteen to twenty years extolling the virtue of music programs designed for older individuals who live both in nursing homes and in the community at large. Many of these articles cite certain aspects of music itself which make it an appropriate treatment medium for

Anne W. Lipe, MM, RMT-BC, received the Bachelor of Music degree in voice performance from Shenandoah Conservatory of Music in 1973. She received the Master of Music from Catholic University in 1975. Her music therapy training is from East Carolina University, Greenville, NC. She has been employed by Asbury Methodist Village as a music therapist for the past five years. She is currently serving as the Mid-Atlantic representative to the Gerontology SubCommittee of the National Association for Music Therapy. Ms. Lipe is currently a graduate student at the University of Maryland pursuing the PhD in Human Development with an emphasis in gerontology. Mailing address: 24724 Nickelby Drive, Damascus, MD 20872.

17

geriatric clients. Kartman (1980) cites the universal appeal of music, and the use of specific nostalgic music as a tool for reaching clients who cannot be reached by other treatment modalities. Palmer (1980) provides an overview of a music therapist's training, and suggests ways in which music can be utilized in treatment of various physical and mental impairments that the elderly face. Articles dealing with the practical aspects of setting up a music program can also be found. Mason (1978) discusses setting up a music program for institutionalized geriatric patients, while Davidson (1980) provides practical guidelines for establishing a community-based music program. Gibbons (1985) exhorts practitioners to provide elderly clients with quality music programs that are challenging and fulfilling.

It would serve little purpose to reiterate once again the therapeutic benefits inherent in music. Other articles in this publication address these benefits, and also provide practical suggestions for implementation of therapeutic music programs in various contexts.

The task of justifying not only music therapy, but other expressive arts therapies as viable treatment media for geriatric clients is indeed a formidable task. In order to address this issue, it is necessary to go further than to simply identify the benefits of music — or any expressive arts therapy — for a given population. The benefits need to be concisely defined and tested using accepted scientific tools and procedures. Dr. Emil Guntheil (1952) has stated that "one carefully observed and recorded clinical fact weighs more than volumes of glib speculation on the value of 'music therapy'" (p. 12). In the area of music therapy and geriatrics, there have been some attempts to do precisely this. Riegler (1980) has compared the value of a reality orientation program with and without music. Her research showed that scores on the Philadelphia Geriatric Center Mental Status Questionnaire improved in individuals who had received music therapy as part of reality orientation sessions. Olson (1984) has measured the effects of player piano music on the elderly. She reported in her study that musical treatment increased physical activity and rhythmic participation, and enhanced positive feelings of well-being. Gibbons (1980) contends that in order to provide musical experiences that match the needs and interests of older populations, it is necessary to determine the musical characteristics present in these populations. Her experimental study indicated that "music activities which incorporate music with marked changes in pitch or duration with simple rhythm patterns should facilitate successful experience" (p. 209). Studies have also focused on identifying a most comfortable loudness level for geriatric patients (Riegler, 1980), and on the assessment of vocal range in geriatric patients (Greenwald/Salzburg, 1979).

To understand the overall benefits of a given therapy is all well and good. However, a general understanding may not be enough to justify the services of expressive arts therapists when dealing with both legislative issues and cost-conscious administrators. As expressive arts therapists, we face a two-sided dilemma. On the one hand, we need to avail ourselves of current methods of evaluation of the effects of our therapeutic intervention on our clients, and develop better methods where existing ones are inadequate. It is necessary that these methods be clear, concise and as scientifically designed as is possible. The development of standard measurement devices is imperative if all expressive arts therapies are to be considered medically necessary forms of treatment, eligible for third-party reimbursement, as opposed to "diversionary," and thus easily accessible to the budget axe. Charlotte Hamill (1980) has defined a therapeutic activity as "one that stimulates changes in the participants' abilities from dysfunctional to functional . . . this process is different from a recreation program where the primary emphasis is on providing pleasure for the participants" (p. 3). Indeed, "diversionary" activities have their place in long term care facilities. However, we need to examine the content of our activities programming to determine what percentage of activities can be classified as "diversionary" and what percentage can be classified as "therapeutic." We need to carefully identify what changes in client behavior can realistically be expected as a result of therapeutic activities, and how to communicate our professional efforts and observations to other health care disciplines.

The other side of the problem concerns itself with the very nature of art forms as therapy, namely, the subjectivity of creative expression. Many health care experts have been working for years to accurately measure aspects of the human psyche such as self-esteem, emotion, and motivation. How an individual responds to a given therapeutic activity will be unique, but it is hoped that patterns of response will eventually begin to emerge which may suggest clues for more than just haphazard application of music or any art form with geriatric populations. We need to encourage the belief among the medical community that in long-term care settings, the absence of pathological conditions doesn't mean that an individual's quality of life cannot be improved.

This leads naturally into a discussion on the place of research. Traditionally, many expressive arts therapists and activities directors have shied away from the areas of statistics, measurements and scientific observation. It is imperative that we develop literacy and skill in these areas so that we can accurately report on what we see happening in our everyday work. Unfortunately, time is also a factor. Many activities personnel wear several hats, and with paperwork, planning, conducting activities, recruiting volunteers, etc., barely have time to become involved with professional organizations, let alone write articles and report observations. Perhaps one solution to this problem would be for activities personnel to team up with students or faculty at local colleges or universities. Let them know what it is that needs to be studied, and work with them to choose and/or develop proper measurement devices.

Laments are often heard among expressive arts therapists regarding the more favored status of physical and occupational therapy within the medical community. One reason for this status is the considerable body of research supporting these therapies. Granted, what these therapies address, namely the development or maintenance of physical, functional skills, is more readily measurable than many of the areas we address as expressive arts therapists. However, that makes our task all the more challenging. We cannot survive as a profession and provide only "diversionary" activities, music or otherwise,for our geriatric clients. It is probably an understatement to say that most activities professionals recognize the therapeutic value in their programs. However, we need to carefully define the parameters of therapeutic intervention, and communicate our professional efforts and observations to other health care disciplines.

Developing a body of literature is a time-consuming, arduous task, but must be done for our professional survival. As the creative arts therapies develop methods to make life better for our older clients, we need to work towards compromise between the benefits of a holistic approach to therapy and the medical-model approach which is the norm in most long-term care facilities. We need to increase our literacy in the hard science areas while convincing those with strictly medical-model approaches that quality of life issues have importance for the long-term care patient.

In the Washington D.C. area, the Music Therapists in Gerontology group has been established to address some of these issues. This group organized over three years ago primarily as a support group and to provide a forum to share information and ideas. So far, we have undertaken two major tasks. First, we have produced a videotape now in the editing stage which highlights the ways in which Music Therapy is applied in our various clinical settings. Our second major task has been this publication. Individual members of the group are often consulted to provide resources or information for other professionals in the field of gerontology. Future projects include (1) Possible coordination with the Montgomery County Science Fair Association to encourage students to consider working on projects dealing with music and its effect on behavior, and (2) coordination with area high schools to orient students to Music Therapy as a profession, particularly in the area of geriatrics.

How to define and quantify "quality of life?" This is the question to which we must address ourselves. Communication among professionals results in new ideas and new hope for old problems. The challenge is ours.

REFERENCES

Davidson, J. Music and gerontology, a young endeavor. *Music Educator's Journal*, 1980, *66*, 27-31.

Gibbons, A.C. Item analysis of the Primary Measures of Music Audiation in elderly care home residents. *Journal of Music Therapy*, 1983, *20*(4), 201-210.

Gibbons, A.C. Stop Babying the elderly. *Music Educator's Journal*, 1985, *71*(7), 48-51.

Greenwald, M.A. and Salzberg, R.S. Vocal range assessment of geriatric clients. *Journal of Music Therapy*, 1979, *16*(4), 172-179.

Guntheil, E. *Music and your emotions*. New York: Live Right, 1952.

Hamill, C.M. and Oliver, R.L. *Therapeutic Activities for the Handicapped Elderly*. Rockville: Aspen Publications, 1980.

Kartman, L. The power of music with patients in a nursing home. *Activities, Adaptation and Aging*, 1980, *1*(1), 9-17.

Mason, C. Musical activities with elderly patients. *Physiotherapy*, 1978, *64*(3), 80-82.

Olson, B.K. Player piano music as therapy for the elderly. *Journal of Music Therapy*, *21*(1). 1984, 35-45.

Palmer, M. Music therapy and gerontology. *Activities, Adaptation and Aging*, 1980 *1*(1), 37-40.

Riegler, J. Comparison of a reality orientation program for geriatric patients with and without music. *Journal of Music Therapy*, *17*(1), 1980, 26-33.

Riegler, J. Most comfortable loudness level of geriatric patients as a function of Seashore Loudness Discrimination Scores, detection threshold, age, sex, setting and musical background. *Journal of Music Therapy*, 1980, *17*(4), 214-222.

Music and Dance:
Tools for Reality Orientation

Alfred Bumanis
Jane Warwick Yoder

SUMMARY. This paper presents a theoretical basis for implementing a music/dance-based reality orientation (RO) program. A scientific study that tests the efficacy of music/dance RO versus traditional RO is described. The results show a nonsignificant increase in orientation in those patients who received music/dance-based RO therapy. Patients with severe Organic Brain Syndrome made fewer gains in reality orientation in both groups, but all members showed substantial social and emotional improvement. Practical considerations and techniques in facilitating music/dance RO groups are given. An attempt has been made to gear this information toward the nonmusician and nondancer.

Reality Orientation (RO) is a method for treating the mentally confused. Traditionally, RO relies upon verbal and visual cues to halt or reverse the confusion exhibited by institutionalized patients. Facts about person, place and time are presented in a classroom setting on a daily basis. This information is reinforced by staff who come in contact with clients around the clock.

Recent trends have indicated the use of a creative arts approach to RO. Weiss (1980) explored the use of art and writing as components of an RO program. Riegler (1980) compared RO programs with and without music. The results showed a significant increase in orientation to the environment in those patients

Alfred Bumanis, RMT-BC, former Director of Music Therapy at Woodbine Nursing and Convalescent Center, Alexandria, VA, is currently a music therapist at the Clifton T. Perkins Hospital Center, Jessup, MD. Jane Warwick Yoder, MFA in dance, is a social worker at Woodbine Nursing and Convalescent Center. She is currently working on her MSW.

23

who received music-based RO therapy. In another research project conducted by Mace and Robins of Johns Hopkins (1985), RO ranked ninth in a rank order list of 10 "Activities Most Successful with Demented Clients." In answers to a questionnaire sent to 346 day care centers for the elderly, sing-alongs were ranked first and physical exercise second as being most successful. The rationale for including music in RO programming rests on the assumption that commitment to music requires reality orientation (Sears 1968). Music provides experience within structure and time-ordered behavior. A person has to be aware and somewhat oriented to participate in a musical activity. Sacks (1985) concludes that the power of music to organize is the characteristic which makes music an effective therapeutic medium.

The link between dance and programmatic RO is not obvious and there is little in the current literature on the subject. Dance therapy is defined by the American Dance Therapy Association as the "nonverbal psychotherapeutic use of expressive movement as a process which attempts to further the emotional and physical well-being, integration and functioning of people" (ADTA 1973). The main focus of dance therapy is to "encourage people to communicate at a nonverbal level, which will lead to verbal discussion" (Burnside 1984). Dance therapy technique encompasses exercise, music, dance, song, touch, structured and improvisational group and individual movement patterns, as well as the use of tactile stimuli and props. It is a broad discipline which can be successfully integrated into the RO technique.

There is support for a connection between various forms of sensory stimulation, mental alertness and the learning process. The "individual suffering from sensory deprivation may give the appearance of a demented state" (Reichel 1980). Damage to sensory cells can lead to a gradual blurring of present reality and self-awareness (Feil 1982).

Dance therapist Eva Garnet writes: "It has been demonstrated in experimental studies that complete sensory deprivation for a period of 30 hours causes hallucination in healthy young athletes. . . . The sensory impairment of increasing blindness, deafness and loss of taste buds, and particularly decrease of the tactile sensations of affectionate relation and loss of kinesthetic sensations for lack of activity, add up to a massive sensory deprivation" (Garnet 1977). The nursing home patient who "has no freedom of access to the world; has no anchorages . . . ; has few cues for orientation; has no variety in the groups with which he may associate . . . " (Gossett 1967) is environmentally deprived of sensory experience. This patient can benefit greatly from a creative arts therapy with an RO approach.

Paradoxically, the confused, agitated patient, unable to focus his attention, may be helped by touch since tactile stimuli can have a calming effect on the nervous system (Ayre 1973); and the lethargic patient may be stimulated and made more alert. There may be a neurological explanation for this phenomenon. Studies have shown that connective fibers extend from sense organs in the brain, up through the reticular or the limbic area and into the cortex, indicating that an activating process may take place when a sensory organ is stimulated. Any kind of stimulation (sensory, emotional, occupational) is helpful, and there is a good possibility that senility can be reversed through it (Oberleder 1969). Music and dance can address the special needs of the institutionalized elderly by supplementing sensory stimulation through modalities that are less impaired and by supporting those that still function.

In order to design an effective RO program which would meet both mental and emotional needs of impaired, elderly patients, an experiment was designed which would compare the results of two different treatment plans. Pre- and post-tests would be given, and descriptive narratives would be written daily on each subject as the program progressed, assessing his or her emotional status. Afterwards, the patients would be placed in a long-term treatment plan based on the experimental results.

METHOD
Subjects

Fifteen geriatric patients at the Woodbine Nursing and Convalescent Center, Alexandria, Virginia, were randomly selected from a list of residents who exhibited a mild to severe degree of confusion, disorientation and memory loss. Subjects were matched according to scores on the pretest and then randomly assigned to experimental and control groups. The mean chronological age of the 2 male and 13 female patients was 81.2 years. The mean chronological age was 67.6 years for the control group, 88.4 years for the RO group, and 87.6 for the music/dance RO experimental groups. Only 4 of the 15 subjects were ambulatory.

Equipment

A blackboard was used for all sessions; this board contained the name of the institution, the day, date, and year. Also used were pictures of the present President of the United States and the President before him. The age and birth date of each member of the groups were also written on the blackboard at appropriate times. The Goldfarb Rating Scale,[1] a test which includes the Mental Status Questionnaire (Kahn et al, 1960) and the Face-Hand Test (Fink et al, 1952) were used as pretest and post-test measures.

Additional equipment for the music/dance experimental group included a guitar, cassette tape player and tapes, rhythm instruments, beach ball, silk scarves, and parachute.

Procedure

As a pretest procedure, the Goldfarb Rating Scale was administered to all subjects. All scoring was completed by the experimenters.

Both experimental groups received an intensive 1/2 hour of classroom orientation daily, 5 days a week. All sessions were lead by both experimenters. Group size was limited to 5 subjects each. The groups met for a period of 2 weeks as recommended in the Guide for Reality Orientation. After the 2-week period, a post-test was administered and the subjects were then placed in a weekly, 1-hour program of music/dance RO conducted as a part of the regular nursing home activity program.

Activities for the sessions included individual reading of the

[1]The MSQ and the FHT are "widely used" (Brink et al, 1979) for determining mental status of confused nursing home patients. The MSQ tests long-term memory, primarily, and the FHT measures sensory memory. In a research study correlating the two tests, the MSQ and FHT had a Pearson Product Moment Correlation Coefficient of .71.

RO blackboard, and reading, writing, and spelling of group members, names, the days of the week, the months of the year, and the ages and birth dates of individual members. Pictures were used in both groups to stimulate discussion. In the music/ dance RO group, each session was centered around a music activity. Rhythm, gesture, touch, and props were used to reinforce the words in songs which were chosen (or composed) to include RO information.

RESULTS AND DISCUSSION

A one-way analysis of variance was conducted to obtain an F score of 1.27. This score was insufficient to reject the null hypothesis at the .05 level. The small size of the groups, the variability of mental capacity of group members, and the short time period of 2 weeks may have influenced the outcome. There was, however, a nonsignificant improvement in all three groups as can be seen in Figure 1.

Merely asking the questions twice seems to have generated some improvement in reality testing. However, it was found that RO presented in a context of multistimuli produced a greater overall improvement than by using visual and verbal cues alone. The music/dance group, which emphasized sensory stimulation, was consistently the most alert and enthusiastic, even though 20 years older on average than the control group. This group also showed greater improvement in social adjustment and in emotional well-being than the other groups. There was greater group interaction and more positive behavior.

We found support for the research of Naomi Feil (1982) in that the better oriented patients did respond and show greater improvement in RO in all three groups. The more severely disoriented residents showed little improvement on the Goldfarb Rating Scale, but did respond to the Validation Treatment Plan which included sensory stimulation, music, and expressive movement. Although the intensive, 2-week program of RO helped the residents by jarring them out of their lethargy and by developing a relationship of trust with the therapists, permanent change did not become apparent until after approximately 6 months of being placed into the weekly music/dance RO program

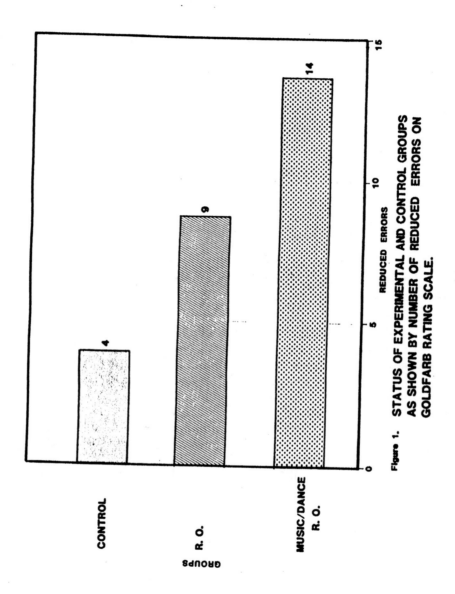

Figure 1. STATUS OF EXPERIMENTAL AND CONTROL GROUPS AS SHOWN BY NUMBER OF REDUCED ERRORS ON GOLDFARB RATING SCALE.

28

provided for all residents. One patient suffering from Parkinson's disease, anxiety and depression showed dramatic improvement 7 months after the experimental program. Since admittance, she had refused to walk unassisted, and withdrew in tears whenever approached. After slowly developing a relationship to the music and dance therapists, she suddenly announced that she wanted to walk. Accompanied musically by the therapists, she began to dance, saying, "This may kill me, but at least I'll die happy!" (Actually, it was just what the doctor ordered.) The floor staff rushed into the room to clap and cheer. The fact that she has shown a slight improvement in RO seemed less important.

PRACTICAL CONSIDERATIONS

Talent

Facilitating a music/dance-based RO program requires leaders who enjoy music and dance, not those who possess great talent. It should be remembered that the leader is not performing for the group, rather that he/she is trying to elicit certain responses. The ability to motivate clients is more important than musical prowess. The music skill most required is being able to sing somewhat on key and carry a tune. If you can get your group to sing along with you, then you have the necessary talent. The same can be said about dance. What is lacking in graceful movement can be made up in energy, enthusiasm and a sense of humor.

Equipment

As for musical instruments to accompany the group, the autoharp is an excellent choice. This instrument is easy for the non-musician to play and is very portable. One drawback is that it is difficult to tune. This problem can be overcome by using an omnichord, a more expensive electronic autoharp. This instrument requires no tuning and some models feature instant electronic transposition. Instruction books and plenty of music are available. A wide variety of portable keyboards are on the market. An electric chord organ can be played with one finger.

A dual-deck cassette tape player is an indispensable piece of equipment. These "boom boxes" are more portable and easier to use than record players, and they afford good sound quality.

Having two cassette decks is an advantage in programming selection. A search feature which helps in locating individual songs is also recommended. A built-in radio can be utilized by tuning in news and weather reports. Headphones and microphones can be used with some models. A Radio Shack store is a good source for customizing equipment.

Selection of Group Members

The study focused on subjects thought to be sensory deprived. In general, those with the diagnosis of Organic Brain Syndrome did not respond as well, but still benefited from the groups. This experiment supported the findings of Naomi Feil. In a qualitative research project, Feil (1982) found that group activities help remotivate disoriented old-old residents, provided that the worker used a nurturing approach. She also found that the oriented residents did respond to RO. However, the more severely disoriented residents showed greater improvement from her Validation treatment plan which included music, movement, and exploring feelings and reminiscing. She found that permanent change had occurred after 6 months. Our experience has been that more oriented individuals are ideal candidates for music/dance RO because results can be objectively verified. We feel that the more disoriented clients do benefit from music/dance therapy, though results are harder to prove.

An assessment of each group member should be made to determine his/her level of orientation. This procedure also helps in developing a treatment plan that focuses on client weaknesses and needs. Groups made up of similar functioning individuals can be formed. The leader can determine which particular areas of reality awareness should be stressed. The Goldfarb Rating Scale and the Philadelphia Geriatric Center Mental Status Questionnaire are assessment instruments which can be used for these purposes.

Ideal group size is five, though a slightly larger group is feasible if there are at least two leaders. A group led by a music therapist and a dance therapist is a luxury. The strength of this approach is that at least one person is free to stimulate, prompt and touch clients. With only one leader, the group size should be limited to five. The 2-week intensive group should always be small.

Place and Time

Treatment groups should emphasize consistency of approach which is found to be the key to the rehabilitation of the confused patient (Guide for RO, 1970). Groups should be held in the same place and at the same time each day. A quiet place, free from distractions such as the P.A., T.V., and other people is required. In addition, the environment should be as pleasant and non-threatening as possible. Our procedure was to place clients in an intensive 1/2 hour per day group for 2 weeks, and then place them in the regular 1-hour weekly music/dance group which stressed RO.

Beginning the Session

An opening/hello song gives a clear indication that the session is starting. The leader should acknowledge each member of the group with eye contact and touch, usually a handshake or a pat on the shoulder. Using each person's name in the hello song helps in motivating the client and reinforces that information for the client and other group members. The ability to use live music is an asset since it gives the leader the flexibility to adapt to each individual.

Any song can be used as a hello song. An example is the tune "When the Saints Go Marching In."

> Oh, When _name_, comes marchin' in
> Oh, When _name_, comes marchin' in
> Lord, We'll all say hello
> When _name_, comes marchin' in.

Clients should be encouraged to suggest and create opening songs. Dance gestures can be added.

Activities

Music and dance activities should be planned for the specific purpose of increasing RO. A multisensory approach using any and all forms of stimulation is advised. Blackboards, mirrors, pictures and other props should be used in conjunction with the music and dance. Improvisational dance or movement can be used to help patients differentiate and express emotions even when they are wheelchair-bound. Therapists can work individually with patients to make a dance by using only the hands. A musician can match the mood and rhythm of a patient and gradually lead him or her into more spirited and expansive movement. The client and dance therapist can focus on mirroring one another.

Well-known songs can be used to lead the whole group in structured dance gestures which reinforce the words of the song. "He's Got the Whole World in His Hands," which is a good opening song, can be used to develop RO for place, person, and right and left hand. As an example:

> He's got the whole world in His hands,
>> (Arms circle overhead and open to sides, palms up)
>
> He's got the whole world in His *right* hand,
>> (Reach overhead with right hand)
>
> Repeat sentence and gesture.
>
> He's got the whole world in His hands.
>> (Clap three times)
>
> Repeat whole verse with left hand.
>
> Repeat verse with *name of place* in His hands.
>
> Repeat verse with *name of patient* in His right hand,
>
> He's got *name of patient* in His left hand, etc.
>> (Shake right hand and then left hand)

As with gesture, song lyrics can be adapted to reinforce basic concepts. The popular song, "Amen," is an example. Information such as name, place, even the main course for lunch can be substituted for the word, "Amen." Thus your group might sing the lyrics, "meatloaf, meatloaf." (This done with a sense of humor, of course.) The simplicity and repetition seem to help the client learn and retain the concept and still make the activity fun. Be consistent in using the same song for the same concept.

Another method of song adaptation is omitting a word and replacing it with one that stresses basic concepts. During "Let Me Call You Sweetheart," the group leader would stop the singing and a client would be asked to substitute his or another person's name. "Let Me Call You *name*." The song, "You Are My Sunshine" can be used to make clients aware of the weather. Our groups have often sung, "You Are My *(Rainy)*." Humor, or the attempt at humor should always be encouraged.

Singing, listening and moving to "seasonal songs" also reinforce basic knowledge. Examples include, "Summertime," "Autumn Leaves," "Winter Wonderland," and " Springtime in the Rockies." These songs serve as a springboard for discussion. Any song whose lyrics relate to the goals of the group can be utilized. Thus "Maryland, My Maryland," and "Carry Me Back to Old Virginia," reinforce concepts of place. Songs should be age-appropriate and lyrics made available in large-type print. The nonmusician has a wealth of recorded material to choose from.

Rhythm instruments, parachutes, beachballs, balloons, fans, silk scarves, and hula hoops can be used to motivate people to move rhythmically to music. A simple parachute dance can be created alternating right and left hands. Beachballs can be tossed among group members until the music stops. The person left holding the ball is then asked a question. Balloons that have information or questions printed on them can be batted around the room. Silk scarves, in various colors and sizes, can also be used as costumes or to wave in time with the music. Many people who feel self-conscious with expressive/creative movement become much more spontaneous and imaginative when given flowing scarves to swirl about them.

Ending the Session

RO sessions should end with a closing/goodbye song. The purpose is to indicate that the session is over. It is a good idea to personalize the song and to make eye contact while singing with them. Touch in the form or a handshake or a backrub is also recommended. The song, "Irene, Good Night," can be adapted to:

> _Name_, goodbye
> _Name_, goodbye
> Goodbye _Name_, Goodbye _Name_
> We'll see you tomorrow!

In closing, it is suggested that professional music therapists and dance therapists be consulted to help in facilitating or designing an RO program for your facility. Qualified therapists might compose songs and prepare tapes which suit specific group circumstances and needs. In-service programs may be arranged and staff instruction provided. For more information, contact the national associations of these professions which are listed in the resource section of this journal. Also, be aware of workshops or conferences which might increase knowledge of techniques, resources and ideas.

There are many intangibles that make RO sessions successful. These include fun, spontaneity and a healthy sense of humor. These areas should not be neglected. Music and dance energize and motivate people. They create just the right therapeutic atmosphere for emotional development, socialization, and learning.

REFERENCES

American Dance Therapy Association. (1973, October). Dance therapist in dimension: depth and diversity. *Proceedings of the Eighth Annual Conference of the American Dance Therapy Association*. Columbia, Maryland: American Dance Therapy Association.

Ayre, J. (1973). *Sensory Integration and Learning Disorders*. Los Angeles: Western Psychological Services.

Brink, T.L., Bryant, J., and Catalano, M.L. (1979). *Journal of the American Geriatrics Society*. 27(3), 126-129.

Burnside, Irene. (1984). Dance therapy. In I. Burnside (Ed.), *Working with the Elderly: Group Process and Techniques*. Monterey, California: Wadsworth Health Science Division.

Feil, Naomi. (1982). Group work with disoriented nursing home residents. *Social Work with Groups, 5*(2), 57-65.

Fink, M., Green, M., and Bender, M.B. (1952). Face-hand test as diagnostic sign of organic mental syndrome. *Neurology, 2*, 46.

Garnet, Eva D. (1977). A movement therapy for older people. In Kathleen Ciddle Mason (Ed.), *Dance Therapy—Focus on Dance VII*, pp. 59-61. Washington, D.C.: AAHPERD.

Gossett, Helen M. (1967, September). *Augmenting and preserving the functioning capacities of aging persons in extended care facilities.* Paper presented at meeting of the Nursing Home Association of San Francisco.

Guide for Reality Orientation. 1970. Tuscaloosa, Alabama: Veterans Administration Hospital, Nursing Service.

Kahn, R.L., Goldfarb, A.L., and Pollock, M. (1960). Brief objective measures for the determination of mental status in the ages. *American Journal of Psychiatry, 117,* 326.

Mace, N., Robins, P. (1985). *Study to identify services day care centers for demented elderly find most successful.* Baltimore: The Johns Hopkins University School of Medicine, Department of Psychiatry and Behavioral Sciences.

Oberleder, M. (1969). Emotional breakdowns in elderly people. *Hospital and Community Psychiatry, 20,* (7), 21-26.

Reichel, William. (1980). The evaluation of the confused, disoriented, and demented elderly patient. *Clinical Aspects of Aging.* Sacks, Oliver. (1985). *The man who mistook his wife for a hat and other clinical tales.* New York: Summit Books.

Sears, W.W. (1968). Processes in music therapy. In E.T. Gaston (Ed.), *Music in therapy.* New York: Macmillan.

Weiss, J.C. (1980). The use of art and writing as therapeutic tools for improving reality orientation. *Activities, Adaptation and Aging, 1*(1), 3-8.

Music and Movement for the Geriatric Resident

Farlee L. Wade

SUMMARY. Music and movement have been closely linked together throughout recorded history. Rarely do we listen to music without feeling the urge to tap our feet, snap our fingers, clap our hands, or to get up and dance. This instinctive urge paves the way for the natural pairing of music and exercise, and is the basis for incorporating movement and exercise. Whether the exercise is the formal structure of "one-two," or the improvisational form of free dance, music enhances the movement. As music therapists, we use music to set the tone and mood for our exercise and dance groups, as well as using such specific music-movement techniques as Rhythm Instruments, Orff, and Eurhythmics. This chapter will present suggestions for adding music to an already existing exercise group, how to set up a music exercise group, how to get geriatric residents dancing; and a brief discussion of each of the above listed music and movement methods.

Adding music to an already existing exercise program doesn't simply mean turning on the record or tape player and using whatever music is lying around. A successful music program reflects careful planning and coordination of the basic elements of the program. Before adding music to an exercise program, the leader should ask him/herself the following questions:

Farlee L. Wade, RMT-BC, graduated from the University of Dayton with a Bachelor's Degree in Music Therapy in 1984 and has had two-years' experience working with the aged in residential facilities. Farlee Wade has worked extensively with Adventures in Movement for Handicapped Children and has adapted many of these techniques for working with the geriatric population. Comments may be addressed to 107 Croyden Ct., Apt. 5, Silver Spring, MD 20901.

1. How long is the group?
2. What type of exercise does the group do?
3. Does the group include a "warm-up" or "cool-down" period?
4. Does the group make use of props such as balls, ribbons, stretch bands or parachutes?
5. What type of music does the group prefer?

The music with which the leader chooses to supplement the exercise program should complement the exercises done. Strong, rhythmic, "calisthenic" type exercises need music with a strong beat to emphasize the repetitions. The tempo (speed at which the beats occur) should closely match the pace with which your residents can perform the exercises. A tempo which is too fast will discourage those residents who are unable to keep pace, and a tempo which is too slow will "drag-out" your exercise program. Free and creative movement can be enhanced by the use of flowing and imaginative music. The music used for warm-up and cool-down movement should be slower in tempo and less strongly rhythmic to help slow down and smooth out the movements of the residents.

Props such as balls, ribbons, stretch bands and parachutes can also provide the basis for successful combination of music and movement. Props can be bought from physical education supply companies, but simple, homemade props, often made by the residents themselves can add an unique dimension to exercise groups. If the exercise leader uses props in his/her group, the music should match the type of movement the prop is designed to stimulate. Ball-tossing (the use of sponge-rubber or yarn balls is strongly recommended for the safety of the residents) to music requires not only the use of arms to catch and to throw the ball, but also requires a certain level of on-task concentration. Calling the resident's name before throwing the ball is a good idea in order to focus the resident on-task. Ribbon waving is a creative movement which allows for self-expression. Satin ribbon approximately 2 inches wide and 24 inches long can be purchased at any fabric store. Asking the residents to "paint" with the ribbon what the music means to them will produce different pictures depending on the music used. A ribbon attached to a length of dowel can become a "magic wand" for either the leader or any member of the group, thus giving the person with the "magic wand" control over what movement the group does. Stretch bands and parachutes can bring a confused or unfocused group together by requiring the cooperative effort of the group in order to move. As with ribbon-waving, faster music will tend to produce faster, jerkier movements; while slower music will tend to produce slower, more flowing movement.

Finally, the music selected should appeal to the residents in the group. This does not necessarily limit the group leader to the music of the 20's, 30's and 40's! Experiment with a wide variety and let the residents choose the music they prefer. The important point to remember is that the music and movement should complement each other, and should therefore be thoughtfully selected. Music with a strong rhythmic beat, such as dance music, is best suited for use with exercises that are rhythmic and repetitious. (See the exercise section of the Sample Exercise Program for examples.) Broadway and movie musical dance numbers, the Big Band "swing" sound, and dance music from any era are good suggestions to get your residents moving. For warm-up or cool-down movement, music which is flowing and creative can help to emphasize the flowing movement needed to stretch gently older muscles and joints. Improvisational piano music, such as that played by George Winston, and ballads from any era are appropriate music for this type of movement. Again, the music and movement should complement each other.

Setting up a music exercise group is a more complex task than adding music to a previously existing group. The same questions should be carefully considered before beginning a music exercise group as well as the following:

1. What type of residents do I want in my group?
2. How big do I want my group to be?
3. How do I want to set up my group?
4. How often do I want my group to meet?

When setting the criteria for membership in the group, the exercise leader should consider whether or not he/she wants alert or confused, ambulatory, wheelchair, or gerichair bound residents. The resident's capability for following verbal direction should also be assessed before admitting him/her to the group. Other important criteria to consider are the resident's attention span and his/her ability to perform the exercises. Multi-level groups can exist, but require a great deal of experience on the leader's part in order for them to work successfully.

The size of the group is dependent on the type of residents in the group and the size of the room in which the group is held. A higher functioning group can be as large as 15-20 residents, while a lower-functioning group that needs more hands-on assistance should be smaller to ensure the success of the group. The room in which the group is held should be large enough to allow each resident room for full range of motion and the group leader access to all the members of the group.

The physical setup of the group allows for several options. Whether or not the residents are placed in a circle, a square, theater or random seating is unimportant. The important thing is to leave enough space to avoid collisions between residents.

The question, "How often do I want my group to meet?," is dependent on a number of criteria. The size of the group, the group's ability to gather in one place (can they all walk there, do some need assistance, is the group leader doing all the gathering, or are other staff members helping?), and the current activities schedule are all factors that should be considered. A small group which is fairly mobile and has a not-too-full activities schedule can meet more often than a large wheelchair-bound group in a crowded schedule that one person has to gather.

By answering all these questions as well as the ones listed previously, the exercise leader can design a group or groups which best suit the needs of the residents. For the beginner, a sample music/exercise program is included at the end of this chapter from which he/she may base the exercise group. It is not intended to be an exact program, but rather a guide for the leader to use when creating his/her group. The primary points for the beginning or advanced exercise leader to remember are to be creative and not to be afraid of experimenting. What doesn't work can always be changed, and the exercise leader may find that as the group evolves it may need change. A group which has been highly structured may find that it needs time to be creative, while a creative group may hit a "dry spell" and need structured movement to rejuvenate its improvisational process.

The most natural form of exercise is dance. Getting the geriatric resident to dance can be both challenging and exasperating. Some residents literally jump right in with both feet, others need to be coaxed, and still others are unable to stand, thus making the traditional forms of dance impossible. Music is often the key motivator in getting residents to dance. A familiar tune from early adulthood can bring back memories of dancing and thus make the resident want to dance.

Dance can be formalized or structured, as in folk and ballroom dance, or improvisational as in modern and jazz. As it pertains to the geriatric population, dance can be defined as the movement of the body to music, either in stylized patterns or in an improvisational manner. Dance is most easily incorporated in the activities program as part of a celebration. Birthday parties, Happy Hours, and seasonal parties are a natural setting for dancing with your residents. Bright and lively music with a not-too-fast beat provides the setting, and a high staff to resident ratio ensures that everyone will get a chance to dance. A two-step around the floor will show other residents that it is still possible for them to dance. Don't forget those wheelchair residents who are weight-bearing with one assist. A nurse or physical therapist can best instruct you on how to dance with them. Often times just providing support under the elbows is enough. These residents are often afraid of falling and need to be gently coaxed into dancing. Take it slowly, step-by-step, and always stop when the resident is ready. That way he/she will trust you the next time you invite them to dance.

Dancing with the wheelchair-bound resident is a challenge. Holding hands and gently moving the arms from side to side is sometimes all the activities a person can do. It is important to include these residents in your dancing. Wheelchair-bound residents often feel left out or forgotten because they are unable to leave the chair without the assistance of others.

For more formalized dancing, or adaptive dance techniques, it is best to consult a dance therapist. Dance therapists are trained in the use of dance and movement as a therapeutic technique, and can easily assist the activities coordinator in designing a therapeutic dance program.

In addition to combining music with exercise and dance, there are several specific music-movement techniques which music therapists use to stimulate movement through music. They are Rhythm Instruments, Orff and Eurhythmics. Rhythm Instruments can be easily incorporated by the layperson into an activities program. Orff and Eurhythmics are highly specialized techniques and are presented for informational purposes. If the activities coordinator or exercise leader wishes to utilize them in his/her facility, a music therapist or other professional trained in their usage should be consulted.

Rhythm Instruments can be purchased through most local music stores that carry school instruments. A good starter set consists of maracas, rhythm bells and tambourines. Instruments should be colorful, lightweight, and durable; handles should be large enough to be fitted into arthritic hands, or be capable of being adapted for the residents. Both exercise groups and sing-a-longs can benefit from the addition of rhythm instruments. Encourage residents to shake the instruments to the beat of the music or to the pattern of the syllables of the words in the lyrics. Having residents shake the syllables of their names to introduce themselves to the group is one way to begin a group using rhythm instruments. As a supplement to an exercise group, rhythm instruments promote creativity and self-expression through movement. Residents can shake the way they feel, the way the music feels, and be encouraged to stretch their range of motion by shaking their instruments overhead, to the right, to the left and down by their feet. Routines can be choreographed using rhythm instruments. The leader is limited only by his/her own creativity and the abilities of the residents.

Orff and Eurhythmics also emphasize creativity and self-expression. Orff, also known as *Schulwerk*, is the invention of the German composer-conductor-educator Carl Orff. Orff believed that in order to learn about music, a person must first feel the music through its most basic element, rhythm. Orff felt that a person was best equipped and encouraged to explore music through the rhythms of speech and movement. Although most widely used with children, Orff techniques can be adapted for use with the geriatric population. *Schulwerk* consists of four phases: the germ idea, development, exploration and closure. It combines learning and easy successful experience to develop communication, sensorimotor, social, and self-help skills. Each participant contributes toward the total, regardless of level of ability. Music Therapists use Orff/*Schulwerk* to stimulate creativity and strengthen the self-image of the participants.

The Swiss music educator, Emile Jacques-Dalcroze, developed the music learning system known as Eurhythmics. Eurhythmics is based on the concept that a person's body is his/her "first instrument" through which a person begins to learn musical ideas. There are two characteristics present in each Eurhythmics session: rhythmic movement and creativity in hearing, comprehending, and interpreting music through movement.

Eurhythmics, like Orff/*Schulwerk*, provides each participant with successful music-movement experiences, as well as the added therapeutic benefits of promotion of attention, concentration, memory, contact with others, balance, coordination of movement, and relaxation.

The benefits of movement for the geriatric person are well known and documented. Physical benefits include increased circulation and lung capacity and improved muscle tone. Social/emotional benefits include increased attention span and memory, improved communication skills, and a more positive self-image. The addition of music to exercise and dance programs can add another dimension to these benefits. Music can provide a stimulating or calming background for movement, and add depth to an existing movement program. The use of props can add an element of creativity, as does the addition of creative dance. Highly specialized music-movement techniques can assist the resident in working towards such specific goals as improved self-image, memory, and communication. Overall, the addition of music can only add to a program of movement for the geriatric resident.

SAMPLE EXERCISE PROGRAM

RESIDENT CRITERIA: Able to follow verbal directions or mimic movement of leader, to maintain attention span of 40 min-

	utes with verbal prompts, to move in both gross and fine motor movements.
LENGTH OF GROUP:	40 minutes
SIZE OF GROUP:	12 Residents
PROPS NEEDED:	Yarn or Sponge Rubber Ball
GROUP SETTING:	In a circle with approximately 1 1/2 to 2 feet between residents.

1. Gather residents for the group. Use music to set the tone for the group. Bright, lively music such as Big Band or songs from musicals is suggested.

2. Greet residents individually. Using the ball, greet each resident by doing individual throw and catch. "Good morning, Mrs. Smith. Are you ready to catch the ball this morning?" Adding a personal comment such as "Your dress looks so good on you," or "Your hair looks so nice today," can aid in focusing the resident on the group.

3. Warm-up. Change the music to a slower, softer tempo to facilitate easy stretching movement. George Winston or other piano improvisations are suggested.

   a. Overhead stretch. Raise arms slowly overhead, stretching upwards toward ceiling. Return arms to resting position in lap. 4-5 times.

   b. Downward stretch. Reach as far down as possible knees, mid-calf, ankles, toes. Encourage resident to go only as far as he/she is able. Return to resting position on lap. 4-5 times.

   c. Neck roll. Tilt head up, right, down, left in a slow circle. 4-5 times.

   d. Shoulder roll. Forward circle 4-5 times; then reverse circle 4-5 times.

   e. Deep breathing. Breathe in through nostrils, out through mouth with a "whoo" sound. 3 times.

4. Exercises. Change the music to a faster, brighter music. Repeat each exercise 10 times to the beat of the music. Take breaks in between movements to allow the residents time to adjust to each movement and to rest.

a. Shoulder lift. Up-down is one sequence.
b. Punching out. Right-left.
c. Punching up. Right-left.
d. Arm Circles. Arms straight forward, small circles inward 10, outward 10.
e. Arm Circles. Arms out to sides, go from small circles to large circles on a 10 count, then reverse the direction.
f. Hand clap. In front.
g. Hand clap. Over head.
h. Knee pat.
i. Swimming. Crawl Stroke.
j. Swimming. Breast Stroke.
k. Rocking. Side to side.
l. Rocking. Forward and back.
m. Toe Taps.
n. Heel Taps.
o. Heel-Toe Taps
p. Kicking from the knee — right then left.
q. Legs apart — together from the knee, meeting at the ankles.
r. Right leg lift. Point toe, flex toe.
s. Left leg lift. Point toe, flex toe.
t. Flutter kick.
u. Cross legs at ankles right over left, left over right.
v. Fist, then stretch.
w. "Windshield Wipers" — move arms from elbows, side-to-side.
x. Wrist circles — move hands in circles from wrists. Forward 10, reverse 10.
y. "Egg Beater" — move hands in circles around each other. Forward 10, reverse 10.
z. Individual. Have each resident contribute an exercise to the group. It may be one already done or a made-up exercise.

5. Cool-down. Repeat warm-up sequence, switching back to slow music. Add:

a. Hand-arm massage. Using one hand, massage arm and hand of opposite side.
b. Neck massage.

   c. Upper chest massage.
   d. Upper thigh massage.
   e. Knee massage.
   f. Calf massage.
   g. Ankle-foot massage.

Some residents may need assistance with these. This is a great opportunity for one-to-one interaction between you and your residents, and also between residents themselves. Encourage more able residents to assist other group members.

6. Closing. Leave on slow music. Thank each resident for coming and invite them to return. Have residents give one final overhead stretch to end the group.

REFERENCES

Gaston, E. Thayer et al. *Music in Therapy*. New York: Macmillan Publishing Co., Inc., 1968.

Geiger, Jo A. *Adventures in Movement*. Dayton: AIM for the Handicapped, 1981.

Needler W., Baer MA. Movement, Music and Remotivation with the Regressed Elderly. *Journal of Gerontological Nursing*, 1982 8(9): 497-503.

Schulberg, Cecelia. *The Music Therapy Sourcebook*. New York: Human Sciences Press, 1981.

Vandevander, E. *Recreational Music*. Class Lecture. Aug-Dec 1981.

"Adding Life to the Place": Musical Activities in the Nursing Home

Michael Lewallen

SUMMARY. A discussion of several musical activities suitable for use with nursing home residents, most of which are geared toward use by activity personnel who do not have extensive musical training. Planning suggestions and instructions for carrying out the activities are included. Specific activities discussed include music listening or music appreciation groups, environmental music, musical games, including music bingo, sing-alongs, resident performance groups, and outside entertainment groups.

Music and musical activities can be of great value and importance to nursing home residents. Music enlivens and vitalizes the environment and provides opportunities for socialization (Alvin, 1975). It can promote social or cultural unity among people who are otherwise strangers by emphasizing their common experience (Alvin, 1975). As a nursing home resident once stated, "Music adds life to the place."

There are so many ways to bring music into the lives of nursing home residents. Different musical activities can be led by people with varying amounts of musical training and ability. The

Michael Lewallen, RMT-BC, holds a Bachelor of Science degree with Honors in biology from Randolph-Macon College in Ashland, VA, as well as a Bachelor of Music Therapy degree with Honors from Shenandoah College and Conservatory of Music in Winchester, VA. He is a member of the National Association for Music Therapy, Music Therapists in Gerontology, the National Association of Activity Professionals, and the American Guild of Organists. He has served as a regional officer in the Maryland Activity Coordinator's Society, and currently serves on the executive committee of the Northern Virginia Chapter of the American Guild of Organists.

major skills needed are enthusiasm, energy, the love of music of any kind, and the willingness to try.

This chapter is for activity professionals and others who want to use music and musical activities to "add life to the place." You will find some ideas, some suggestions, and some things to consider when planning a musical activity. This is not, indeed could not be, an exhaustive resource. Not all programs will work in every facility. You know your residents, their experience, interests, and capabilities. You also have many creative ideas of your own — don't be afraid to try them. And remember, if an idea doesn't work, either your own, mine, or anyone else's, then try it another way, or try something else. Do whatever you can to keep your "creative juices" flowing — your residents can only benefit.

I will discuss several types of musical activities in varying amounts of detail. These will include music listening and music appreciation groups, environmental music, musical games, sing-alongs, resident performance groups, and outside entertainment groups. First, however, some general considerations should be mentioned.

The foremost consideration in planning *any* kind of activity is to *know your residents*. How long is their attention span? What are their cognitive skills? Physical capabilities? Musical interests and abilities? Probably more of your residents enjoyed or performed or participated in some kind of music-making than you might realize. Whether as concert violinists, or church choir members, or virtuoso "radio players," most of your residents have made music a part of their lives in some way. Find out how. Another important bit of information is the residents' cultural background — ethnic origin, religious background or affiliation, education, and geographic location. These factors affect the musical experience and knowledge of the residents and should be taken into account. As an example, consider one nursing home located in a rural, mountain community and another located in an affluent metropolitan suburb. Residents at the first nursing home are likely to have grown up with and participated in bluegrass music and Protestant hymn singing, while residents at the other facility might be devotees of opera and the symphony. There is certainly nothing wrong with playing either kind of music for either group — indeed, variety is encouraged — but it is important to know the residents' musical background. Know their musical "home."

Next, what kind of experience are you trying to create? Purely social? Popular, familiar music, or exposure to "new" things? Active participation or passive observation? Each of these has its place, each should be included in your program at some point.

What is the target population for the activity? Is the activity geared towards alert, oriented, active, highly functional individuals? What about the less oriented or extremely confused? Probably all of your residents can enjoy some kind of music on some level. Not every resident will be able to participate in every activity. Do try to have some kind of musical experience for everyone as part of your overall program.

MUSIC LISTENING/MUSIC APPRECIATION GROUPS

Both of these groups involve listening to music, usually recorded music, as the primary activity. The two terms, music listening and music appreciation, are often used interchangeably. Music is listened to and enjoyed as a pleasant experience, and can also be a vehicle for learning, growing, and expanding one's experience.

What do you listen to? Music the residents prefer is the obvious starting place. You will have some ideas, based on your knowledge of your residents. When in doubt, ask. Some of your residents will certainly be able to tell you what they know and like. Do not be dismayed if what they like is not what you like. (If it isn't, that doesn't prevent you from playing your music from time to time — just don't neglect their preferences.) Also, be aware that the preferences of the groups as a whole may not be quite the same as those expressed by the few most vocal residents. You can try different kinds of music and note which your group responds to. Play a variety of music over a period of time, both for its own sake, and possibly to meet the needs of those nonvocal members of the group whose preferences may not have been expressed. You can have general music listening groups in which a wide variety of music is played, or groups which focus on a specific type of music — show tunes, bluegrass, or opera, for example. Seasonal, cultural, or religious observances can suggest material for your group—for example, Christmas music in December, patriotic American music in July, gospel music or jazz in February (Black Awareness Month). Use your imagination!

Before setting up your group, decide upon the mode of participation you desire from the residents. Will the group involve active listening, listening with a specific agenda, or discussing the music afterwards? Will the group involve passive listening or listening for enjoyment only? Do you want to structure the group as an educational experience? What do you wish for the participants to accomplish? This could be as comprehensive as a survey of Western music or the history of jazz, or learning about musical instruments, or famous tenors since Caruso. It could be as simple as listening to something out of the ordinary once in a while. The residents may have specific ideas—ask them.

When setting up a music listening group, try to find a room with good acoustics and with minimal distractions. Your facility may or may not have an "ideal" music listening room—you might have to try a few locations to see which works the best. Ideally, the room should not have heavy carpets and draperies, as these soak up sound. Lobbies or other areas which have a heavy flow of traffic should be avoided, if possible. But if you don't have an "ideal" place to listen, listen where you can.

There are several ways to present a music listening program. One is simply to tell the group what you are going to play, and then play it. Other methods of presentation involve commentary or discussion about the music. The group leader or a knowledgeable resident could provide information about the music, the performer, or the composer. The plot of a musical or opera could be outlined. The group can discuss the music, what they heard, how it made them feel, or of what images or events they were reminded. The discussion could be guided before the music is played, e.g., "Listen to this music and tell me what instrument is featured," or "Why does this music remind you of Christmas?," or "Be prepared to describe the music in two or three words." The music could be presented in conjunction with some other type of information or program—for example, a series on astronomy involving pictures and information about our solar system, along with selections from Holst's "The Planets."

Where do you find music to play? Most nursing homes have a stack of old records hidden around somewhere — take a look and see what's there. If you have recordings of your own, use them. Borrow from friends, go to the library, ask other staff members and volunteers. Sometimes the residents or their families have recordings they will allow you to use. If your budget will permit, buy some records or tapes, especially if multiple uses are possible. A recording of "Oklahoma" for your music group could then be used another time as background music during a party or happy hour. Always be on the lookout!

ENVIRONMENTAL MUSIC

I am using the term "environmental music" to include several types of music used predominantly as background music within a facility. Such music can be used for a variety of reasons, and should be evaluated on the basis of your facility's needs and the music's effectiveness.

Probably the first things most people think of when they see the term "environmental music" is "Muzak." "Muzak" is the trade name of a specific company which produces specialized prerecorded music for use in work settings, offices, hospitals, and so forth. "Muzak" is technically a registered trademark specifying the product of the Muzak company, although the name is commonly (and incorrectly) used to indicate any kind of "piped-in" music. Some companies provide radio music rather than specialized prerecorded programming.

Music played throughout a facility is a mixed blessing. It can contribute to an overall pleasant atmosphere in the nursing home; however, it may be agitating to some residents, or tranquillizing to others. It must also be controllable; you must be able to turn it off in rooms where programs occur. Trying to speak to a group, or listen to music, or watch a movie can be extremely frustrating if the background music cannot be shut off in that room. Also, residents with some hearing impairment, especially those who wear hearing aids, may not be able to sort out the background music from the other sounds around them.

There are times when background music is quite beneficial. Soft music in dining rooms or other patient areas during mealtimes can stimulate appetite and aid digestion (Lundin, 1967). Music enhances the social aspects of mealtime and stimulates conversation and interaction among residents. It is also beneficial to have music playing before a large group activity. If music is playing when residents arrive for an activity, they become less bored while waiting for others to arrive; this is especially important in facilities where transportation takes a long time. People who are less bored before a function begins seem more likely to stay awake and alert during the program. Conversation is stimulated, as no one needs to feel inhibited about breaking the silence. The music can also be used to "set the scene" for the activity to follow—for example, a recording of Irish songs before a St. Patrick's Day party, or the soundtrack of a Fred Astaire musical before a movie.

MUSICAL GAMES

There are any number of musical games which can be played by the residents. One important factor to consider when choosing such a game is age-appropriateness. Some of the musical games found in resource books are geared towards children and must be adapted for use with adults. Even when working with regressed residents, materials should be adult in nature and then adapted for lower functioning individuals as needed.

Some of the most popular musical games involve recognition and recall of melodies and song lyrics. They can be structured in several ways to suit the number and abilities of the participants. Some considerations: Will the games be played by the group as a whole, by teams, or by individual players in turn? Will scores be kept? Will prizes be awarded, and to whom? Is the game all-in-fun, or is competition encouraged? You might want to try intramural competition between floors or units, or competition between nursing homes. I suggest playing games "for fun" the first few times you try them so that participants won't be intimidated, and so you can see what modifications need to be made to fit your specific situation before competition rules are "carved in stone."

"Name That Tune" is a game which many residents will enjoy. The ability to play piano or some other melodic musical instrument is helpful, although not absolutely necessary. There is likely to be some resident, volunteer, or other staff member who could play the melodies if needed. Songs can also be taped ahead of time, although you have far less flexibility when using pre-recorded music. The basic game is simple — all or part of a melody is played, and participants must guess the title of the song. You may want to allow commonly known first lines as well. The group can then sing the song, if desired. Use a variety of songs, but emphasize those familiar to the residents in order to ensure a successful experience for them. You could organize your selections around a theme if you wish — holiday songs, or songs with colors in the titles, for example — but a good mixture of songs always works.

One variation on "Name That Tune" involves recalling song lyrics. The first line of a song is presented, with or without the tune, and the participants must provide the second line. Or conversely, the second line could be given, and the participants must supply the song title or first line. Yet another variation would be to give a phrase from within the song, for which players must give the song title. An example of this would be to give the phrase "the rockets' red glare," for which the players must respond, "The Star-Spangled Banner."

Another musical game which the residents are sure to enjoy is Music Bingo. I wish to acknowledge the invaluable information regarding this game provided by Millie Becker, whose excellent discussion on handbell groups is found elsewhere within this volume. Music Bingo, some call it "Singo," is an enjoyable activity for the participants, combining song recognition, the element of chance, and a little healthy competition. However, this activity requires a bit more preparation than many others, mostly to make the equipment prior to playing the game for the first time.

The first task before playing Music Bingo is to make the playing boards. Decide how many squares will appear on each board. Twenty-five squares, as in regular Bingo, works for alert, mostly oriented groups. Once you have decided upon the number of squares per board, choose the number of songs in your "song pool." This should be a few more than the number of squares on the playing board — perhaps thirty songs for a twenty-five square board. It is important to realize that playing tunes and giving song titles takes considerably longer than calling numbers. If you have too many more songs in the pool than you have squares on the boards, the game will be very long, and the players will be likely to lose interest. Next, make a list of songs for your "song pool." Your list could be thematic if you wish, but a variety is probably best. All songs used in the game should be familiar to the players — again the admonition, "Know your residents!"

The next task is to put the song titles in random order on the playing boards, realizing, of course, that every board will not contain every song. Possibly the easiest way to make each card different is to put standard bingo calling numbers, one for each song on your list, in a bowl or bag. After numbering the songs on the list, pull numbers out of the bag to determine to order of songs on each playing board. Note that this procedure must be repeated for *each* playing board you make.

Music Bingo is played much like regular Bingo — a song is played, and players who have that song on their board mark it with a token. The player who gets five in a row (or whatever pattern you decide) wins. But where do the songs come from? There are several possibilities. If you play piano by ear, or know the songs on the guitar or autoharp or can play them on the kazoo, you're home free. Play the songs in some random order, keeping track of which ones you've played; making a deck of file cards with one song on each card works well. What if you don't play by ear? You can always sing the songs unaccompanied. You can also put together a little booklet with the tunes written out, or with copies of the music. If you do this, remember to play the tunes in random order, using your deck of file cards, or whatever. Don't just play the songs in order from your book — you'll get the same songs in the same order every time. Even if none of these options is possible, you can still play the game. Find someone to play the songs for you, and make a tape recording. This is the least preferable means of providing the songs, but it works when no other avenue is available. Have your song-provider play through the list twice, in a different order, placing each series on the opposite side of a cassette tape. This gives you two different song sequences right from the start. To make additional sequences, start either side of the tape at some point other than the beginning. If you do that, and you reach the end of the tape before someone wins, rewind to continue with the first song on the same side, otherwise you'll get songs duplicated within the same game. Now you're ready.

I'll admit that the initial preparation and making all the equipment is time consuming and somewhat tedious, but after the initial outlay of time and materials, there is very little preparation necessary for play. Your residents will enjoy it — it's worth the effort!

A few tips for playing the game are in order here. First, have plenty of helpers to assist the players. Because song titles are longer than two-digit numbers, the print in each block on the playing board will be of necessity smaller than that on a standard Bingo board. You might wish to avoid singing complete songs, just giving enough of each to be recognized. Singing complete songs may make the game go on too long, but if the players *want* to sing every song, why not?

Music Bingo can also be adapted for use with more confused residents. Since attention spans are shorter, boards with fewer squares are called for — perhaps ten, or six, or even three. Also, you can use the same number of songs as you have squares, so that each song appears on every board.

SING-ALONGS

Sing-alongs are a valuable part of an activity program. Residents are able to enjoy them on a number of levels, whether through active participation or by observation. Of course, the idea is to encourage as much active singing and participation within the group as possible, but don't overlook those individuals who cannot or choose not to sing along — they can derive much benefit from the activity on their own level.

The key to a successful sing-along is a good leader. This is someone who is energetic, unself-conscious, and capable of motivating the group to sing along. The leader needs to be able to carry a tune recognizably, but is *not* necessarily the person with "the best voice." In fact, a leader with a highly-trained singing voice sometimes seems to inhibit participation—everyone would rather listen. Enthusiasm is important—if the leader doesn't seem to be enjoying the songs and the people, no one else will; enjoy!

Some sort of accompaniment is generally desirable, but is not absolutely necessary. For instance, a group of residents carolling for roombound residents at Christmastime can be very successful. A strong leader can carry a group without accompaniment if need be, but the accompaniment really does add a lot of support. Enthusiasm, unself-consciousness, and energy are important characteristics of a good sing-along accompanist—you must be able to play your instrument smoothly enough to support the singing, with the ability to keep right on going when mistakes are made. If you don't fall apart because of a few "clinkers," no one else will even notice.

It is also possible to use pre-recorded music as accompaniment. Mitch Miller's many records, or the sing-along cassettes available through Presta Sounds (see the Resource List) are good sources for this. While live accompaniment is best, pre-recorded accompaniment is a good alternative. The major drawback to pre-recorded sing-along music is that your program is pre-determined and is far less flexible. Spur-of-the-moment changes based on your perception of the mood of your group and their responsiveness are impossible. You also need to have access to several sing-along recordings if you don't want every program to be the same.

What do you sing? When in doubt, ask the residents. Perhaps you could get their suggestions in advance to allow time for preparation. "Old favorites" which are known to the majority of your group are always a good idea, but remember that "old favorites" can vary from group to group. If you play by ear or have several songbooks, you can always take requests. Another alternative is to choose songs based on a particular theme—seasonal songs, hymns, or songs with people's names in the titles, for example. If you choose a theme, decide beforehand how you will deal with requests for songs that don't fit into your scheme. Will you sing them anyway, or promise to include them another time?

Preparation is important. Decide approximately how many songs you will sing, then prepare twice that number. Depending on the amount of participation, your original list may fly by. Even if you are doing a program "by request," have a list of songs ready in case no one requests anything. It happens sometimes, and there's nothing like standing in front of a group of people trying to think of songs to sing to make you forget every one of the hundreds of songs you know. Having a long list of songs from which to choose also enables you to be more flexible. Suppose you have a list which includes several peppy, up-tempo numbers as well as ballads and love songs. If your group likes both kinds that day, wonderful! But if your room is hot, or everyone is tired, and peppy songs just don't work, you already have alternative music planned.

What about printed lyrics? They are not necessary if you are doing very familiar songs, but can be quite helpful. Song sheets or booklets are one possibility; lyrics printed in large letters on a flip-chart are another. If you use songsheets or booklets, have extra helpers on hand to help everyone keep their place. Having staff members, family members, or volunteers present to sing along, clap, and help keep the group energy up is also helpful.

Sing-alongs can be tremendous fun—just plan, be enthusiastic, and enjoy. It is important to realize, however, that just as with any other kind of activity, there will be times when you are exquisitely prepared and fairly bubbling over with confidence and enthusiasm, and the sing-along just dies. There are many contributing factors. Is the room too hot and humid? Or too cold? Does everyone have the February rainy-day blahs? Is the percentage of active, alert, participatory residents within your group too small that day? Is the resident with the strongest voice at the beauty shop? Are the participants seated too far apart, or too far from the leaders? *Don't give up*. Try to analyze what happened, *ask the residents*, and then see if the particular problem can be corrected or allowed for next time. Keep trying. A sing-along that "clicks" is really a wonderful thing, lots of fun for all involved.

PERFORMANCE GROUPS

There are several types of performance groups in which residents can participate. This discussion will include some basic remarks, and will then focus on choruses. Rhythm bands and handbell choirs are discussed elsewhere in this volume by Farlee Wade and Millie Becker, respectively, and instructions for organizing a variety show can be found in *Accent on Rhythm*, by Donna Douglass (see Resource List.)

Why have a performance group in the first place? Such a group can serve a number of functions and have a number of benefits. It can be an outlet for active residents with musical backgrounds to continue participating in an activity which is important to them. It can be a way for residents to do something for someone else, which is important for maintaining feelings of usefulness and self-esteem. It can foster a sense of group identity, both in the sense of the residents belonging to the group, and in the sense of the group representing the residents of the nursing home as well. The performing aspect of the group is important — it gives the group a reason to exist and provides the reason for residents to participate.

How is the group selected, and who is appropriate for the group? There are several ways to choose the participants. The first, and probably the most threatening, is for residents to gain admission to the group through audition. Using this method is likely to scare away most potential participants before you start. Another method is to make the group open to anyone who wishes to participate. Using this method will almost certainly net a few individuals who attend faithfully, but actually participate very little, if at all. You must decide whether this is acceptable or not. You, as the leader/director, can invite residents to participate based on your knowledge of their capabilities — for example, you might approach those individuals whom you see participating enthusiastically at sing-alongs or other musical functions. Another factor to consider is the visual acuity of potential group members. Will reading songsheets be required? Is there a place for those individuals who might not be able to read the words of the verses, but who join in with gusto on the more familiar refrains? No matter what the selection process used, you might hear comments from some participants regarding other individuals whom they feel do not belong. Be prepared to defend your selections.

Group identity is important. Perhaps the group could choose a name for itself, or a theme song with which to open or close rehearsals or performances. Suggestions for these should come from within the group, not from the leader.

The reason for the performing group is to perform. A long-term goal might be for the group to perform in the community, perhaps at a nearby church, or even at another nursing home. To begin with, the group could perform at various functions within their own facility—a few songs at a birthday party, patriotic songs for the Fourth of July, or Christmas carolling in the halls for shut-in residents. The group's performance could be part of a staff/resident/volunteer variety show. The performance itself might be a "gift" on behalf of all the residents in the facility— for example, a performance as part of a program at a volunteer recognition or staff appreciation function. After they have performed in front of other people a few times, the group will probably be anxious to perform whenever they can.

As an example of how the above ideas work in a concrete situation, consider the chorus at Sleepy Hollow Manor Nursing Home in Annandale, Virginia. The chorus was organized about two years ago. Initial participants were gathered by open invitation as well as by personal invitation to a few individuals previously noticed in sing-alongs. Chorus members sometimes suggest the invitation of new residents whom they hear at church services or musical activities. Songsheets are used by most of the participants, but most of the songs are familiar. Rehearsals are held weekly for one-half hour. A period of at least six to eight weeks is allotted in the preparation of any program which consists of approximately six songs. This period of time allows the group to become thoroughly familiar with the songs, and gives visually impaired and mildly confused residents who do not use songsheets a number of opportunities to become familiar with the lyrics and music. The group has performed at several facility functions, including parties, variety shows, and volunteer recognition functions. Plans are being made for the group to perform away from the facility within the next year. The group sings in unison for all performances at present, as the individuals who can easily sing harmony have the strongest voices and are heavily relied upon by others in the group. Various participants sing short solo parts in performance—for example, the verse preceding a more familiar refrain, which is sung by the entire group. Participation in the group has been very enthusiastic, and the members of the group are always asking when they can perform again.

Performance groups can be an exciting addition to a facility's program. They require considerable planning, and require a leader with a strong musical background, but can be very meaningful and enjoyable for the participants.

OUTSIDE ENTERTAINMENT

Another way to "add life to the place" with music is through the use of outside entertainment, i.e., not otherwise affiliated with the nursing home. Bringing music from the community into the nursing home is of double benefit—it provides enjoyable musical experience for the residents and provides a link between them and the large community of which they have been a lifelong part.

There are several sources of entertainers which should be investigated. Churches and schools usually have choirs or other performing groups. Perhaps you have musicians among your friends and acquaintances. Surely your residents or their families know of musical groups or individuals. Do not be afraid to ask colleagues at other nursing homes whom they use or assist your local activity association in compiling a list of local entertainment resources. Sometimes your volunteers will find entertainers for you. A terrific example here—a group of volunteers from my facility went to a restaurant, where they heard a piano player they enjoyed. They asked him if he had ever played at a nursing home before, and now he comes to the facility at least once a month, at no charge! You may get people from the community who call and offer their services to entertain the residents. This one is sometimes sticky—you very often have only their word as to their competence. I'll usually give them a try. If they're good, so much the better. If not, well, they probably won't get invited back. Subscribe to the local, community-oriented newspaper — through their notices you'll learn of groups within the community of which you might not have been aware.

What types of entertainment are appropriate? Virtually anything, keeping in mind the residents' preferences and the benefits of providing variety. The season or occasion might suggest some possibilities, as do your budget and the availability of various types of entertainment in your area.

Once you've booked someone to entertain, and your residents like them and want them to return, how do you get them to come back? It is important to make the experience of coming to the nursing home as pleasant as possible for the entertainers. Make sure there is someone, perhaps a resident, to greet the performers when they arrive. Keep your piano tuned and in good working order if you use performers who play or accompany others on that instrument. Find out ahead of time what is needed for space, seating, equipment, a glass of water, or whatever else you might be required to provide. If the person or group has never performed in a nursing home before, or has never even been inside one before, you might consider not including the very confused, noisy, and disruptive residents in the activity. Above all else, say "thank you" at least "two hundred seventeen" times. Send a thank-you note, or better yet, have a resident send a thank-you note, even if you had to pay for the performance.

ONLY A BEGINNING

One more word. The emphasis in this chapter has been on music *groups* of different kinds. Please don't neglect the bed-bound, or extremely confused, or socially isolated residents who cannot, will not, or perhaps should not participate in group activity. Take music to them. Sing songs at their bedside, or play recordings of their favorite music. Anne Lipe's chapter on Music Therapy as a one-to-one activity offers many good ideas — see which ones work for you.

This chapter has been essentially a list of suggestions for getting music groups started in your facility. Choose what you will, try what you will, change what you will. Your efforts will really pay off in "adding life to the place."

REFERENCES

Alvin, Juliette. *Music Therapy*. New York, Basic Books, Inc. Publishers, 1975, 88.
Lundin, Robert W. *An Objective Psychology of Music*. New York, The Ronald Press
    Company, 1967, 319-321.

English Handbells
in Nursing Homes

Millie Becker

SUMMARY. English Handbells can add a meaningful adult level musical activity to the program of a nursing home. This article contains practical ideas and helps for starting a bell program in your facility.

English handbells have been one of the more successful educational and recreational musical tools to be used in recent years. Their popularity can be measured in part by the fact that there are thousands of groups of all ages actively ringing in the United States. This popularity is due to the beautiful tone quality and great enjoyment of playing them.

I was both excited and apprehensive upon learning that our Nursing Center was planning to purchase a set of English hand bells. Not only were the residents unfamiliar with them, but my sole exposure to bellringing occurred when a handbell choir performed at our church.

I quickly discovered that while there were articles available describing the use of English handbells with mentally retarded children and adults and even with the blind, nothing dealt with

Millie Becker served as a church organist for thirty years in various cities on the East coast. She developed many unique opportunities to enhance her natural musical abilities during a fourteen year period in Norfolk, VA while singing and creating background music for three syndicated radio broadcasts originating there.

The author began working with the elderly in 1977 and joined the activity department of Fairfax Nursing Center as their music specialist shortly after moving to northern Virginia in 1978. In addition to weekly piano/organ entertainment and sing-a-longs, Millie provides vocal and autoharp music for the roombound residents. She is a certified Activity Director and is presently the Assistant Director of Activities and Coordinator of Volunteers at the Center.

the needs and challenges of handbells with the handicapped elderly. My only clue was a short paragraph I had read in a newsletter about a nursing home in another state whose residents played bells by number. It was apparent that I would have to devise a system of adapting to the unique problems of our residents, all of whom suffered from varying degrees of physical or mental disabilities.

English handbells are still uncommon or even rare in long term care facilities for the elderly. While this is due in part to budgetary considerations, it is more likely that the many benefits and rewards of a handbell program for both the resident and the facility needs to be explored and understood.

HOW HANDBELLS BENEFIT THE RESIDENT

Physiological

- Maintains alertness, concentration and manual dexterity
- Restores left-to-right progression
- Develops eye-hand coordination
- Reinforces exercises learned in physical and occupational therapy
- Aids in relearning old motor skills

Psychological

- Provides an additional key to motivation
- Increases self-confidence
- Develops a new sense of self-worth
- Produces a feeling of being needed
- Encourages socialization
- Provides a new avenue of enjoyment
- Gives an opportunity for musical participation and achievement
- Gives a sense of purpose and pride in belonging
- Develops responsibility and commitment

Handbells Benefit the Facility

— Enhances the quality of the activities program
— Raises the visibility of the facility in the community (especially true when a group is developed which performs outside the facility)
— Opens opportunities for interaction and involvement with community groups, churches, etc.

WHY HANDBELLS?

One very important concern of the activity department in long term care facilities is the need for a balance between active and passive activities for its residents. With handbells, each ringer must "do" to make the sound. Individual as well as group cooperation is required. Unlike rhythm band instruments or melody bells, English handbells produce a type of "instant beauty" even when a simple melody is played. Bell ringing is an adult, sophisticated and dignified activity with wide appeal to residents of varying physical and mental abilities. Those with a musical background and good rhythm are excited about being able to maintain their level of interest and participation in music and it is a thrill to those who never dreamed of being able to "make" music.

HOW TO START A HANDBELL PROGRAM

Get Ready . . .

Introduce Handbells to Your
Administration and Residents

1. Schedule a handbell concert at your facility. Call local churches. If they have a senior citizens handbell group, that is preferred. Ask them to share some things about handbell ringing with the residents.
2. Invite someone from Administration to be present.
3. Observe the level of resident interest.

4. Request permission to have a representative of one of the handbell manufacturers come and demonstrate their bells.
5. Encourage some "hands on" experimentation with the residents.
6. Discuss benefits to the resident and facility with Administration.
7. Discuss the lifetime investment for the relatively small cost and ways the funds could be generated for your facility. A handbell representative can help with fundraising ideas. (See appendix)

Staffing Needs

1. Director (Qualifications)
   A. Staff member or volunteer. (A member of a local handbell choir may be willing to do it.)
   B. Should be able to read music and have a good sense of rhythm.
   C. Must enjoy working with handicapped adults.
   D. Must possess patience.
   E. Prior experience with handbell ringing helpful but not essential.
2. One assistant is adequate if the group is alert and oriented.
3. It is essential to have two assistants if the group is more physically or mentally impaired (i.e., new stroke victims, Alzheimer's Disease, etc.).

Equipment Needs

1. Handbells
   A. Basic Set—25 bells. (Two octaves)
      (1) New—(see appendix)
      (2) Used
         a. Classified ads of a newspaper.
         b. Classified ads of *Overtones*, the magazine of The American Guild of English Handbell Ringers (see appendix).
         c. Post a notice on the bulletin boards of several large churches with handbell choirs.
      (3) Borrowed—a local church may be willing to loan

some of their bells which are not being used, or share their bells with you on days they are not using them.

(4) Many simple tunes can be written for as few as eight bells.

2. Easel
   A. Large and sturdy enough to support standard size poster board used for charting music.
   B. Tubular light attached to the top of the easel to make the charts more visible to the residents.
3. Music Charts
   A. 16 × 22 inch heavy white poster board
   B. Heavy black marker for preparing charts
   C. Pointer
4. Washable white gloves (available through handbell suppliers)
5. Tables
   A. Any available tables could be used initially with foam for padding.
   B. Folding tables approximately 16" wide and 6' long (permanently padded) are ideal. (See appendix)
   C. Make your own tables by purchasing sturdy steel folding legs. Cut plywood to desired size. Cover and staple padding over the plywood.

Resident Ringers

1. Guidelines for selecting *primary* candidates
   A. Former musicians or those keenly interested in music
   B. A good sense of rhythm (helpful but not essential)
   C. Reasonably good eyesight
   D. Enough strength in one arm and hand to hold and ring the bell (bells vary in sizes and weights)
   E. Adequate alertness to follow simple directions
   F. Adaptability to change
   G. Appropriate social behavior
2. Guidelines for *secondary* candidates
   A. Those needing a graded activity to improve:
      (1) Attention span
      (2) Endurance

(3) Gross motor coordination
(4) Upper extremity strength
(5) Cognitive functioning (ie. time, place, purpose, sequencing, memory)
(6) Self-esteem
(7) Social behavior
B. Those needing an opportunity to interact with and encourage residents having similar disabilities.
C. Visually handicapped, blind or deaf residents.
D. Residents with severe mental impairment. (Mental *dis*ability does not mean *in*ability).

Get Set. . . .

Adapting the Music

1. Decide which charting method to use. This will be determined by the residents who will be participating.
2. Some charting options
   A. Musical notation (for high level, former musicians) (See Figure 1)
   B. Note letters (See Figure 2)
   C. Numerals (See Figures 3 and 4)
   D. Colors (See Figures 5 and 6)
   E. Other symbols
3. Music Selections
   A. Prepare several simple exercises or songs using the symbols selected. A simple melody line from a songbook can be copied, assigning numbers, colors, etc. for each bell.
   B. Several songs requiring only six or eight bells:
      (1) Old MacDonald
      (2) Mary Had a Little Lamb
      (3) Three Blind Mice
      (4) Are You Sleeping?
      (5) Good Night Ladies
   C. Select songs which are familiar to the residents in order to make the rhythm easier to follow.
   D. Music charting assistance is available. (See appendix)

ARE YOU SLEEPING

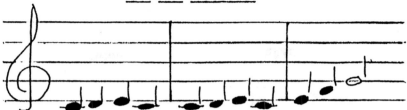

Figure 1. Musical notation

ARE YOU SLEEPING

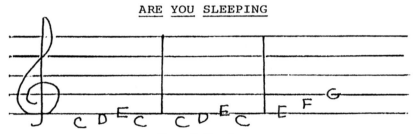

Figure 2. Note Letters

ARE YOU SLEEPING

6-8-10-6   6-8-10-6   10-11-13

Figure 3. Charting by numerals

ANCHORS AWEIGH

6-10-13-15-10-15   18-20-13-18
6 - 10 - 10   13-17-11-13
6 - 6   10-13-8-10
5 - 3   6-11-5-6
                        1 - 8
                        5
                        1

Figure 4. Charting by numerals

OLD MACDONALD

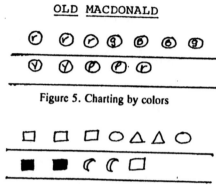

Figure 5. Charting by colors

Figure 6. Charting by colors

Adapting the Bells

1. The bells should be marked to coordinate with the charts.
    A. A small sticker with the number, symbol or color can be placed on the bell handle.
    B. Colored yarn can be tied to the handles if color charts are used.
    C. Special mallets for striking the bells are available if residents are unable to lift or hold the bells (see appendix).

Go!

Time to Ring

1. Seating arrangement
    A. The open U seems to work best, placing the easel and music in the center.
    B. Residents are seated according to visual needs, ability to concentrate, wheelchair space and sometimes temperamental considerations.
2. Washable white gloves should be worn to protect the lustre of the bells and give a more uniform appearance (especially when performing.)
3. Frequency and length of sessions
    A. Weekly sessions are ideal in order to maintain continuity and remembrance.

B. Begin with thirty minutes and increase to one hour as resident interest and endurance develops.
4. Pointing or cueing options
   A. With an alert group, point to the notes or symbols from left to right in the rhythm of the song.
   B. For less alert residents, set up a large placecard in front of each person with their number or symbol on each side. (Provides a cue for the director and ringer.)
   C. If residents are too visually or mentally impaired to use charts, simple melodies can be played by pointing directly at each person when it is his/her turn to play. Use placecard with this option.
   D. If the resident is blind, a volunteer or alert resident can stand or sit behind the ringer and tap them or gently squeeze the shoulder when it is their turn to ring.
   E. Since color charting seems to work best for residents with Alzheimer's or other related mental disorders, a square of fabric or felt with the assigned color can be placed in front of each person.
5. Ringing the bells
   A. Keeping the same bell assignment for each person helps to develop a greater degree of confidence and proficiency.
   B. Each ringer may be responsible for one or more bells, depending on individual ability or choice, as well as the melodic importance of certain bells and the frequency with which a given one must be rung.
   C. For the benefit of those with the use of only one arm, it is important to assign bells that do not often ring in sequence.
   D. Demonstration of holding and ringing techniques should be reviewed at each session.
   E. Chart some simple scales or the Westminster Chimes in several keys to aid in reinforcing each resident's assignment.
   F. Limit verbal instruction. Remember the Chinese Proverb:
      What the human hears is soon forgotten . . .

What the human sees is remembered . . .
What the human DOES is understood!

Confucius

G. Always reward their efforts with smiles, compliments and encouragement.

EXPANDING YOUR HORIZONS

A Personal Word

It has been seven years since English handbell ringing was introduced to the musical/activities program of our facility. At the time, we had a number of residents who showed a keen interest in the idea of bell ringing, having been exposed to some small toned bells by a former volunteer.

After acquiring our own set of 25 Schulmerich English Handbells, the hard work began. It took weeks of discouragement and defeat coupled with excitement and enthusiasm to work out methods of picking them up, holding them and determining the bell weight each person could manage. Often we had to start all over the next week due to personal setbacks of group members or even death. At times I doubted we would ever be able to play a recognizable song, but the determination and commitment of the residents, as much as my own, eventually came to fruition.

As we progressed and began to produce pretty music in two, three and even more note chords, I decided the group needed an opportunity to perform. Our first outing was to provide the entertainment for a Christmas party at a local church. We watched the residents have their hair done, make arrangements with families for a white blouse or shirt to wear and nervously count the days and hours. The enthusiasm with which we were received brought tears to our eyes. A new dimension for life and living was being reborn in these people to replace the feeling of worthlessness. This group continues to do community performances once or twice a month. Our own lift-equipped van is used to transport the residents and equipment.

By then, other residents were becoming interested in trying to ring the bells. Since the maximum number for seating and manageability was twelve, an intermediate group was formed. These residents started with the basics and progressed gradually to the level of the advanced group. As their abilities increased, they became backups for the first group and candidates for a permanent position.

A therapy group was organized shortly afterwards with the help of our occupational therapist who assessed and recommended residents she felt would benefit from this type of rehabilitative involvement.

It has only been a short time, at this writing, since we began trying the bells with residents having Alzheimer's Disease or more severe mental impairments. We are encouraged by the response thus far. One woman (a former member of the advanced group) no longer recognizes her own family and is often unable to feed herself. Yet, when given the same bell that she used to ring, rarely misses a cue.

One of many success stories which inspired us was that of a 34 year old woman who was staying at our facility for one year following an automobile fire accident. Severely scarred and suffering the physical and emotional effects of brain damage and partial paralysis, Sue's activity involvement was nil. Even the small problems encountered in her daily A.D.L.'s were overwhelming and brought on a barrage of tears. As a friendship developed between us, and after much coaxing, she agreed to try the bells. It was only a short time before Sue was sitting before audiences, assisting me in the setting up and taking down of equipment and recruiting others for the group. Now, some four years later, she is completely rehabilitated, living in her own apartment in another state and is volunteering in a facility for the handicapped. She has told me many times that her involvement with bell ringing here was the first step in accepting her limitations and realizing that a fulfilling life was possible.

I remind you that this has all happened over a period of years. There are no overnight miracles. But I do promise you the reward of seeing your bellringing residents personify hope and inspiration to the other residents in your nursing home as well as to correct the misconception that a nursing home is a "place to die" rather than live a meaningful life.

The opportunity and challenge are ours!

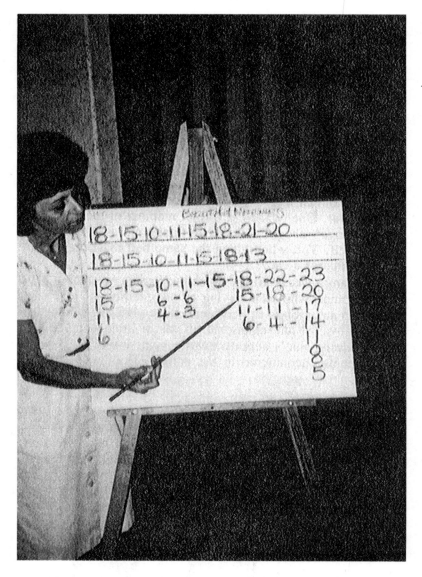

Photo 1. Director Millie Becker with music chart for advanced group

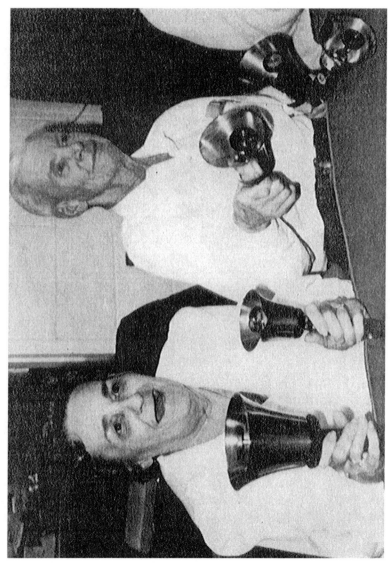

Photo 2. Mae Silzle and Walter Lund, Fairfax Nursing Center

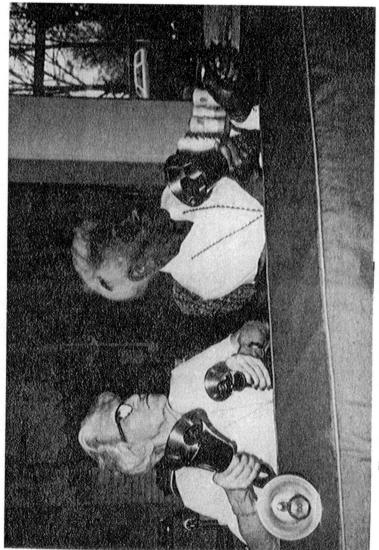

Photo 3. Rose Blumenthal, age 92 (left) and Rosa Lewis, age 98, Fairfax Nursing Center

76

Appendix

Sources for New Handbells

Bissell Handbell Supply and Services
2734 Wrexham Ct.
Herndon, Va. 22071

Rod Davis Music Co., Inc.
2549 Forest Drive
P.O. Box 4275
Columbia, S.C. 29240

Schulmerich Carillons, Inc.
Carillon Hill
Sellersville, Pa. 18960

Whitechapel Bell Foundry, Ltd.
34 Whitechapel Rd.
London, E1   1DY
England

Malmark
21 Bell Lane
New Britain, Pa. 18901

The Handbell Connection
1032 Redondo   Box 91235
Long Beach, Ca 90809

Used/Reconditioned Bells

Classified Ads of Newspapers

Overtones Magazine
601 West Riverview Avenue
Dayton, Ohio 45406

Miscellaneous Supplies and Equipment

Bissell Handbell Supply & Services
(see above)

Rod Davis Music Co., Inc.
(see above)

The Handbell Connection
(see above)

Jeffers Handbell Supply, Inc.
Carillon Park   Rte.2 Box 159
Irmo, S.C. 29063

A.G.E.R.
National Headquarters
601 West Riverview Avenue
Dayton, Ohio 45406

APPENDIX, continued

Music Charts   (Notation, numerals, letters, colors, symbols)

Millie Becker
Fairfax Nursing Center
10701 Main Street
Fairfax, Va. 22030

Music and Reminiscence:
For Groups and Individuals

Beckie Karras

SUMMARY. This article includes background information on the use of reminiscence in a geriatric setting. Practical suggestions are given on how to successfully use reminiscence and music as valuable therapeutic tools with both groups and individual geriatric clients. Personal reminiscence examples are included.

What comes to your mind when the word "reminiscence" is said? You may envision the large porch of an old frame house in the country. Three rocking chairs are softly moving in the lazy afternoon heat. Who are in the chairs? Old people, of course, with maybe a youngster there, too, daydreaming while they talk. For most people, reminiscing implies old age, though we all reminisce.

Thirty years ago, many clinicians considered reminiscence to be a useless preoccupation with the past and even harmful to one's mental health. In 1963, Dr. Robert Butler, then a resident psychiatrist at the National Institute of Mental Health, wrote an influential paper on life review. He concluded that there was "a universal occurrence in older people of an inner experience or mental process of reviewing one's life; that it helps account for the increased reminiscence in the aged, that it contributes to the occurrence of certain late-life disorders, particularly depression,

Beckie Karras, RMT-BC, is a 1973 graduate of East Carolina University in Music Therapy. She has worked as both music therapist and activities director in Maryland nursing homes for the past ten years. She was a co-founder, with Louise Lynch of the Washington, DC area Music Therapists in Gerontology. In 1985, she authored *Down Memory Lane*, a program book for doing reminiscence groups with seniors. Mailing address: 11821 Idlewood Road, Wheaton, MD 20906.

and that it participates in the evolution of such characteristics as candor, serenity, and wisdom among certain of the aged" (Butler).

Life review is a natural process to older people; perhaps because they are facing the ends of their lives or perhaps because of changes in the realities and importance of time and memory in the brain. Many older people need to put some order to the past as well, to make some sense of it.

Memories often come crowding back to an older person. One spark will set the whole mind whirling into another time and place. And the face will get a certain glow to it, one of faraway concentration, as the person relates what is remembered, as clearly as if it were yesterday.

Here is one person's reminiscence, "sparked" by the song "Alice Blue Gown":

> I remember a song called "Alice Blue Gown." When I was five my mother made me an Alice Blue gown. My mother made all my clothes.
>
> I went to Georgia Avenue to the little store Seigworth and I bought Alice Blue ribbon with my own money. I wore my Sunday shoes and marched down the street just all dressed up. I was at a military installation, now the Veterans Hospital. I think the soldiers liked to see the girls all dressed up.
>
> This was before blue jeans. When we wanted to relax, we wore bloomers instead. They were government issue with buttons down the front. I wore them to my gym class.
>
> *Dorothy Ahrens*

Reminiscence groups can be of particular benefit to older people. Not only is there pleasure in remembering and relating the past, but there is joy in sharing with those who have lived through the same times. They feed each other's memories and give each other recognition for past accomplishments. At times there is shared sympathy at a tragedy of the past. Reminiscence groups can also help overcome the loneliness and separateness so commonly felt by residents of nursing homes.

How does a group leader evoke these memories? It is difficult to predict what the spark will be that will cause a group of older people to reminisce together. When leading a group on "Hometowns" once, I began asking questions about the stores they used when young. Suddenly, everyone began talking at once, naming stores, what they had bought there, and the exact location in the city. One woman lovingly described a hat that had been specially designed for her at a local shop.

There are dozens of props that can be used to encourage this kind of reminiscing — antiques, old photographs, scrap books, food, films, vintage clothing, and . . . music!

Why use music? First, it is an excellent way to create an atmosphere of the past. It sets the stage, so to speak, for a bygone era and its attendant memories. Music has been recorded all through this century. The wide appeal of the Victrola insured that all generations born in this century grew up with music surrounding them, making it a universally shared part of the culture.

Second, music not only arouses memories of the past, but also feelings about the past. Can you remember a lullaby sung to you as a child? If so, you will probably also remember who sang it to you and how you felt about that person. Finally, music is enjoyable, a good motivator, and helps create a nonverbal bond between people.

Before undertaking a group, it will be helpful to know about the background of the participants. To begin, you may want to screen the members of your group. People who are aphasic may or may not want to be a part of it, depending on how frustrated they become when unable to share their own thoughts. Many Alzheimer's patients cannot participate because their memories and their ability to communicate are too impaired. It is sometimes better to have the more confused or forgetful residents in a separate group so that they are not intimidated by those who may have very extensive recall of the past. However, memory is unpredictable. I have been surprised many times at the memories related by someone who can't remember that she finished breakfast five minutes before.

Your group will run easier if you know something about your participants' past lives; for example, who was married, where they grew up, what kinds of jobs were held. It will also help if you can learn specifically about the years in which your group was young, especially the teenage and young adult years. Check out *This Fabulous Century* from the library and look through the many pictures and short articles that describe life in the United States during each decade. Knowledge of historical facts alone isn't enough. Note how life has changed, what the culture was like, who the heroes were, what daily life was like, what songs were popular. You can learn much of this from the residents, but some foreknowledge will go a long way in encouraging them to share with you.

USES OF MUSIC IN GROUP REMINISCENCE

My interest in reminiscence began simply because I wanted to try something new at our facility and I have a personal interest in oral history. At the first group session, which I called "Down Memory Lane," we talked about fashions of the past, using a list of clothing terms. The residents of the nursing home were so enthusiastic that I scheduled another group soon afterwards on the topic "Hollywood." Gradually, a format evolved from the groups and I began to make extensive use of appropriate objects and music. One woman rarely talked during the group meetings but always stopped me afterwards to relate a memory and say "That 'Memory Lane,' I like that."

The following ideas have been successful in using music to encourage reminiscence in groups:

1. Music can be played in the background as the group members gather, to set the mood for what is to come. It's always fun to use particular songs that enhance a topic, e.g., playing railroad songs if you're going to discuss trains or transportation. I have found that people don't usually pay close attention to specific songs while gathering and socializing, but instead pick up the mood. For that reason, it is just as useful to play any music that they would have heard when young, e.g., dance music of the 1920s, songs of Fred Astaire, or Glenn Miller's orchestra, depending on the era you are going to discuss. It is important to use the *original* recordings for this. These can be found at estate sales or libraries, or purchased through companies specializing in nostalgia music, such as Prestasounds. (See the Resource List.)

2. Music can be used as the topic for a reminiscence group; for example, "American Popular Song," "Music In Our Lives," "Singing Stars of the 1920s," "Music and Dancing," or "Opera." With many appropriate musical examples, you can focus in on their experiences with music and how it touched their emotions and, perhaps, affected their lives.

3. Many topics for reminiscence groups lend themselves to using groups of songs on that topic. Here are some examples:

— Weddings . . . love songs ("I Love You Truly").
— Vacations . . . songs about places ("Alabamy Bound").
— Fashions . . . songs mentioning clothing ("Alice Blue Gown").
— Pets . . . songs about animals ("Old Grey Mare").
— Mothers . . . songs with women's names ("Ramona").

Ask the residents to name all the songs they can remember on your topic and sing some of them together. You could also play "Name That Tune" by playing a song, letting the residents guess the title, then singing it together. It's helpful to prepare a list for yourself in advance. Look through the index of a songbook (pre-1950s songs) to find some titles. (Lists are also available in the book *Down Memory Lane* by the author, as well as other resource information for reminiscence groups.)

4. Another way to use topic songs is to focus on songs and their lyrics. The song "Five Foot Two, Eyes of Blue" mentions "turned down hose" and "flappers." After singing or listening to the song, you can talk about fashions of the 1920s or what it was like to be a flapper. The song "School Days" mentions writing on slates. Some of the people in your group may have learned to read and write that way and will tell you about it. Many old songs mention other images from the past that you can use for discussion. Here are some examples:

— "Meet Me In St. Louis" . . . state or world fairs.
— "Sidewalks of New York" . . . how do you "trip the light fantastic?"
— "10 cents a Dance" . . . have any ever danced for money?
— "You Must Have Been a Beautiful Baby" . . . beauty contests.

— "Jingle Bells" . . . using a "one-horse open sleigh."
— "In My Merry Oldsmobile" . . . early cars.
— "Bicycle Built for Two" . . . marriage proposals or bicycle riding.

5. I like to start and end groups with an appropriate song, one that is very familiar to those in your group. For example, a group on "Friends" could use these songs:

— "Make New Friends"
— "The More We Get Together"
— "Getting to Know You"
— "Give My Regards to Broadway"
— "Auld Lang Syne"

6. For the music to be effective, the songs used in reminiscence must be ones that the residents know from the past, especially their teenage and young adult years. A song that would be inappropriate for the group on "Friends" is the Beatles' song "With a Little Help From My Friends." However, you can use more recent songs (though sparingly) as a basis for talking about the past. Write the words in large print and give a copy to everyone before you play the song. Here are some songs that could be used this way:

— "Those Were the Days" . . . for a discussion of friendship.
— "Sunrise, Sunset," from "Fiddler on the Roof" . . . for a discussion of weddings or of children growing up.
— "Old Time Radio" by Garrison Keillor . . . for a discussion of radio.
— "Get-Up-and-Go" by Pete Seeger . . . for a discussion of growing older.

7. Another way to use lyrics in a group is as a means for moving into a more serious topic. This should be done with only a very small group whose members are familiar with each other and communicate well. Hymns are an excellent choice for initiating discussion on religion or of life and death. "Brother, Can You Spare a Dime" could start you on the Depression. "Keep

the Homes Fires Burning" could focus your group on the war years. These topical areas, however, can evoke very strong feelings; music can be a very potent force. Unless you are trained in how to deal with expressions of strong emotions, I would caution you to steer away from these kinds of discussions. Certainly, any topic can bring memories that will cause someone to cry. You may find you need to consult your social worker if something seems to be especially painful to someone. But deliberately probing into events that were very traumatic in someone's life can do more harm than good and you can very quickly get in over your head. In my groups, I don't avoid emotions, but I do seek to keep the discussion light, lively, and moving.

8. One activity that has been particularly popular among reminiscence groups is identifying singing voices. Artists such as Bing Crosby, Kate Smith, Eddie Cantor, Billie Holiday, Fred Astaire, Al Jolson, and Louis Armstrong have distinctive voices and styles. Play an excerpt from one of their songs and ask the group members to guess who is singing. This can be followed with a discussion of the song, the singers, or of the year or era; add pictures if you have them. A related activity is to name or to play famous theme songs and have the residents name the singers known for these songs. Here are some examples:

— "When the Moon Comes Over the Mountain" . . . Kate Smith.
— "Thanks for the Memories" . . . Bob Hope.
— "Thank Heaven for Little Girls" . . . Maurice Chevalier.
— "Over the Rainbow" . . . Judy Garland.
— "Stormy Weather" . . . Ethel Waters or Lena Horne.
— "Take the 'A' Train" . . . Duke Ellington.

9. Another group of songs with many possibilities are those with historical significance. This could be a topic for a group by itself or used as history comes up in other discussions. Here are some examples:

— World War I—"Over There" or "How Ya Gonna Keep 'Em Down on the Farm."
— Franklin Roosevelt's theme song—"Happy Days Are Here Again."

— World War II — "God Bless America," "Don't Sit Under the AppleTree," or "I'll Be Seeing You."
— Roaring Twenties — "Charleston" or "Ain't We Got Fun."

10. If you ever go browsing in used book stores or in antique shops, look for original old sheet music. These are a real treasure. They can be used first as just a visual prop — something to remind people of the past. Second, the pictures on the front and the song titles are often useful for starting discussions. Here are some choice ones that I've found:

— "Faded Love Letters of Mine," 1922 — The cover shows a group of letters tied with a ribbon, sitting on a table beside a beaded lamp.
— "Thanks for the Buggy Ride," 1925 — The cover shows a man taking his flapper girl friend out for a buggy ride with a very spirited horse leading the way.
— "The Desert Song," 1926 — The cover shows a sheik carrying away a wide-eyed girl (reminiscent of Rudolph Valentino).
— "When We Sang That Song of MOTHER Then I Thought of Home Sweet Home," 1918 — The cover has a photograph of an aged Victorian woman, complete with wire-rimmed glasses, a lacy blouse, and a cameo pin.
— "Oh! Frenchy," 1918 — The cover shows a nurse with one hand on the shoulder of a soldier and her other hand touching her heart.

A third use for original sheet music is with the verses to the songs. Many times these verses will reveal a historical bias that the chorus doesn't have or they tell a story that makes the chorus more meaningful. I had thought that "Sleepytime Gal" was a trite, sexist, 1920s song; however, the verses tell of a young man whose girl friend wants to go dancing every night until 2:00 a.m. while *he* wants to go to a movie and get to bed early for a change. In the chorus he dreams of the day when they can settle down as married people and get to bed by 8:00. He's dating a happy flapper and she's wearing him out!

"MUSIC AND MEMORIES":
AN OUTLINE FOR A GROUP SESSION

Topic: "Sweethearts" (for St. Valentine's Day)
Opening Song: "Let Me Call You Sweetheart"
Name That Tune: Play or sing some of the following songs that have the word "Heart" in them and have the group guess the titles. Or, ask them to name songs that contain the word "heart."

—"Heart of My Heart"
—"The Gang That Sang 'Heart of My Heart'"
—"I Left My Heart in San Francisco"
—"Let Me Call You Sweetheart"
—"Peg O' My Heart"
—"Goodnight, Sweetheart"
—"Sweetheart of Sigma Chi"
—"Sweetheart" ("Will You Remember")
—"My Sweetheart's the Man in the Moon"
—"My Heart Stood Still"
—"Heart and Soul"
—"Young at Heart"
—"Two Hearts in 3/4 Time"
—"Zing! Went the Strings of My Heart"
—"Hard-hearted Hannah"
—"With a Song In My Heart"

Discussion:

1. "Ain't We Got Fun?"—What did a couple do together to have fun?
2. "After the Ball" or "Sleepytime Gal"—What kinds of dances were popular for couples?
3. "O Perfect Love" or "I Love You Truly"—What music was used at weddings?
4. "It's Been a Long, Long Time"—Who remembers their first kiss?
5. "Baby Face"—Who can remember pet names used by you or your sweetheart?

6. "When You Wore a Tulip" — Do you remember sending or receiving flowers?
7. "Yes Sir, That's My Baby" Does anyone remember their marriage proposal?
8. What are your favorite love songs?

Closing Song: "Goodnight, Sweetheart"

USES OF MUSIC AND REMINISCENCE WITH INDIVIDUALS

If you have the time to do some one-to-one life review, many of the previous suggestions can be adapted. However, this setting gives you more opportunity to discover the place of music in each older person's life. Specific songs can be discussed in depth, using lyrics as cues, and you can learn more about the feelings behind events in their lives. As mentioned before, it is essential that you use the music of their younger years.

Many excellent books exist on taking life histories. One I recommend is *How to Tape Instant Oral Biography* (Zimmerman). It can be read quickly and has specific questions and ideas about doing life review. There is also a bibliography available from the American Association for Retired Persons that lists many books and articles on the subject of reminiscence (AARP, 1909 K Street, NW, Washington, DC 20049).

The following are music-related questions that can be used in individualized sessions:

1. What is your earliest memory of music in your life?
2. Did you have a player piano in your home? Did you have any other musical instruments in your home?
3. Did your family have a regular singing time?
4. What music do you remember from your church or synagogue?
5. Did you have music in school?
6. Did you ever study music?
7. Did you ever take piano lessons?
8. Do you remember going to band concerts?

9. Did your parents ever take you to hear an orchestra or a concert by a famous musical artist or star?
10. Do you like to sing?
11. What is your favorite song?
12. Did you and your spouse have a special song?
13. What music did you use at your wedding?
14. What did you sing to your children?
15. Who was your favorite singer? Did you ever see him/her in person?

REMINISCENCES

A song can bring back some very special memories. There is a great variety in response to reminiscing to music. The following three "reminiscences" were shared by residents of a nursing home as part of a writing group, led by teacher Mary-O Steinwinter. The theme for the group was "Songs I Remember."

My mother, the mother of seven children, and a farmer's wife, needless to say, spent a hard working life. There were so many chores. But she was always singing, as she walked around the house. We learned the 23rd Psalm from her daily repetition as she walked around the house, with a bright light reflecting in her eyes, accomplishing her daily chores. Then I remember the song she would sing at Christmastime:

"Santa Claus brought me a dolly,
And the eyes are oh so blue;
And she goes to sleep so jolly,
Don't you wish you had one, too?"

Of course, all this I can recall and repeat on my head computer anytime I so desire. We have much to be thankful for.

Eleanor O'Brien

I can't sing! For some reason I can't "carry a tune," as the saying goes. When my son was little and I would attempt to sing, he would look at me imploringly and ask, "Mother, must you?'' Then one of my grandsons, age four or five, asked me, after we had all joined in singing "Down By the Old Mill Stream" while driving home from the beach, "Grandmother Vida, why can't you sing good?" But in my mind's ear I sing beautifully with never a sound to be criticized. One of my earliest songs of memory is "In the Shade of the Old Apple Tree." I remember playing with my sisters and singing this song in the shade of a "board ark" (bois d'arc) tree in our back yard and imagining (and wishing) the bois d'arc tree was an apple tree. Other songs I've loved and remember are "Over the Waves," which my father played on his harp, and "Stumbling," which my husband and I danced to on our honeymoon at the St. Francis Hotel in San Francisco, nearly sixty-four years ago.

Vida Hickerson

Since I've never had an ear for notes, my own singing has always wavered, but my soul can sing when I hear great voices. Even remembrances of special songs give beauty that becomes almost visual. I remember a performance of "Tristan and Isolde" at the Met with Helen Traubel who was an enormous woman matched by Lauritz Melchior. But he was suddenly ill and replaced by a too-small-to-match tenor. Last minute changes caused havoc on stage and the audience had reason, frequently, to laugh at a slipped up wig, a ridiculously mismatched love scene, and badly aimed sword play. Tragedy became farce. It was awful! Then came the final scene when Isolde cries out her terrible grief. Miss Traubel defied the still tittering audience and seemed to shrink to the scared teenager she was supposed to be as she poured out her soul in the "Liebestod," as I'd never heard it sung before. I reached out for my husband's hand, thinking her voice could have been mine if I had lost him. When the time did come so many years later and my grief was great, it was her lament so long ago silenced that sobbed through the silence that was mine.

Helen L. Anderson

CONCLUSION

Reminiscence is a nearly endless subject and one that has myriad possibilities for exploration. Music, as an integral part of our culture, adds a dimension of feeling that increases the value of the experience for nearly everyone. You will find, too, that it is not only beneficial to the people you serve, but will enrich your life as well.

REFERENCES

Butler, Robert N. "The Life Review: An Interpretation of Reminiscence in the Aged." *Psychiatry, Journal for the Study of Interpersonal Processes*, 26 (February, 1963) 65-76.

Karras, Rebecca. *Down Memory Lane, Topics and Ideas for Reminiscence Groups*. Wheaton, Maryland, Circle Press, 1985.

This Fabulous Century. New York: Time-Life Books, 1970.

Zimmerman, William. *How To Tape Instant Oral Biography*. NewYork: Guarionex Press, Ltd., 1979.

The Use of Music Therapy as an Individualized Activity

Anne W. Lipe

SUMMARY. The nursing home will always contain individuals who require individualized activities programming. Most often, these individuals will be those who are severely impaired in both cognitive and physical functioning areas. Music provides an excellent treatment medium for these individuals for a variety of reasons. Music sessions for these individuals can be presented through the use of tapes or live music. When possible, live music is preferred because of the increased possibilities for both personal interaction and spontaneity. Individual music visits should be structured, and should utilize goals and objectives for the individual's responses which are compatible with levels of functioning. Those residents who have exceptional music talent or training may also require individualized programming to provide challenges or encourage leadership roles.

In nursing homes, there will always be residents who require individualized programming. Reasons may include: severe mental and/or physical impairment, confinement to bed, tendency to be disruptive in groups, severe confusion, or self-imposed isolation due to actual or perceived impairment, or lack of social skills. There may also be residents in these facilities who have exceptional ability or background in a given area and thus require

Anne W. Lipe, MM, RMT-BC, received the Bachelor of Music degree in voice performance from Shenandoah Conservatory of Music in 1973. She received the Master of Music from Catholic University in 1975. Her music therapy training is from East Carolina University, Greenville, NC. She has been employed by Asbury Methodist Village in Gaithersburg, MD as a music therapist for the past five years. She is currently serving as the Mid-Atlantic representative to the Gerontology SubCommittee of the National Association for Music Therapy. Mailing address: 24724 Nickelby Drive, Damascus, MD 20872.

more challenge than can be offered through traditional small or large group activities. There is some mention in the literature of the need for individualized programming, and what forms this programming might take. Bright (1972) emphasizes the importance of stimulation for the bed-bound, and asserts that in some ways, their needs take priority over the needs of those who can walk. Foster (1980) stresses the need for individualized activities. She states that "if the need for individual activity is not addressed, the incidence of social isolation within the facility is increased" (p. 36).

Music provides an excellent medium for individualized programming. Music has a wide appeal and one can either be an active participant or a listener. Most people can relate music to certain life experiences, which can encourage reminiscence. The great variety of musical styles allows for programming that will fit the needs and interests of almost any individual. Discussing music can open channels of communication and even the severely impaired can respond to the rhythm in music. Hymns often provide a link between past and present, and can provide spiritual affirmation for those attempting to find meaning in their lives and prepare for a peaceful death. Music can also serve as a reality orientation tool in that participation in music activity takes place in the here and now, and demands time-ordered behavior (Gaston, 1968).

In discussing the use of music in individualized programming, it is necessary to consider two general populations. First, those who are severely impaired in both physical and mental spheres, and who are generally confined to bed. Often, these individuals are unable to communicate verbally, and are those who require extra creativity on the part of activities personnel in providing them with mental and social stimulation. Because they are generally unable to advocate for themselves, they are often left alone in their rooms with blaring TVs and radios for companionship. Human companionship is what is needed for these residents, along with extra reassurance that they are special and worthwhile as human beings. These are individuals whom volunteers will often shy away from either because of lack of social feedback, lack of skill in knowing how to work with them, or for fear of becoming like them.

How can music benefit these people, and what forms should music intervention take? The need to discontinue use of TV and radio as a constant stimulant cannot be emphasized enough. Even if family members have requested and provided radios and TVs for these residents, their use needs to be monitored. In cases where recorded music is desired, it would be advantageous to take the following steps: (1) research the resident's history, and where possible, consult family members about music preferences, (2) make or purchase tapes which include these preferences. If it is not possible to obtain preferences, include a variety of selections when making a tape. Include some up-beat selections such as "Roll out the Barrel" ("Beer Barrel Polka"). "Just Let a Smile be Your Umbrella," or "I'm Looking over a Four-Leaf Clover." To ease tension and anxiety, include some waltzes such as "Waltz of the Flowers" from the *Nutcracker Suite* or some of the popular waltzes of Johann Strauss.

Quiet hymns can also be effective in promoting a decrease in anxiety. This is because hymns are easily recognized by these residents, and have the ability to provide an immediate focus for attention. One particular recording that I have found useful is "A Time of Peace — Ivory Sessions" (Maranatha! Music, P.O. Box 1396, Costa Mesa, California 92628). Nostalgic favorites from the 1890s, the turn of the century, 1920s and 1930s may also be well-received depending on the ages of the residents involved. Patriotic songs, too, are usually favorites. It might be advisable to have several tapes available, each devoted to one of the above categories. Playing a tape will provide a structured way for a volunteer to visit a severely impaired or bedridden resident. Guidelines and supervision of volunteer visits could be structured by professional activities personnel, and visits could be discussed to provide helpful assistance with interpersonal techniques. Providing this type of structure might assist in alleviating burnout and allow a positive experience to develop. Such tapes could also be used by other staff. For example, tapes could be loaned to nursing staff to play when a resident is particularly anxious, and activities staff may be busy with other duties.

The vital element in individual programming is the personal contact. For an individual visit, select an area that is quiet and free from both auditory and visual distraction. When initiating a visit, tell the resident who you are and why you are there. Remind the resident what type of day it is. Touch frequently, and comment on musical selections. In the case of a nonverbal resident, encourage reminiscence by statements such as "perhaps you can remember when . . . " instead of using questions which the individual may be unable to answer. Always treat the resident like an adult, and assume that he/she can hear and understand, even if he/she may not be able to give a verbal response. Avoid terms of endearment.

Whenever possible, live music may be preferred over recorded music. This is because live music is more personal, and allows for greater variety and spontaneity. In my work with the severely impaired, I use an autoharp because of its small size, and the fact that I can play it easily. An Omnichord II is also a useful tool for individualized programming. Any individual who chooses to use an instrument such as the autoharp, guitar or ukulele must have good command of the instrument so that the focus of attention during a session can be on the resident and his/her responses. If live music is planned, make sure that keys to songs are comfortable for both the musician and the resident. I try to pitch keys from the g or a below middle c to the c or d one octave above middle c. As to length of time for individual sessions, or frequency of sessions, use the resident's needs, interest and level of functioning as a guideline. I usually make individual visits once a week for about 15-20 minutes. Based on the assumption that increased contact might increase levels of response, twice a week sessions may be preferable.

With the severely impaired resident, look for responses compatible with the resident's level of functioning. A response to music might include spontaneous eye contact, body movement, tapping of fingers or clapping of hands, attempts to communicate verbally, or facial expressions. Responses may also include attempts to hum or sing along with the melody. It may be necessary to visit a resident for several sessions before observable responses occur. Naomi Feil in her book *Validation-Fantasy Therapy* offers many helpful suggestions for working with the severely disoriented. Her suggested techniques can be easily incorporated into individual music sessions.

Individual music sessions might also benefit those individuals who cannot participate successfully in groups due to severe confusion, communicative disorders or behavioral problems such as heightened anxiety or agitation. For these residents, music can provide a reality-based focus for attention, or it can be paired with exercises to promote relaxation. Recordings from the Windham Hill label may be helpful in working with these residents. After assessing a resident's level of functioning, establish one or two realistic goals and objectives for individual sessions. For example: *Goal*: "increase attention span through twenty minute individual music sessions × 2 weekly." *Objective*: "Resident will attend thru eye contact with therapist to _____% (identify percentage of time) of session within _____" (identify period of time for achievement of this goal).

Another group of individuals within the nursing home setting who might benefit from individual music programming are those who have a strong background and/or exceptional talent in music. Since these individuals may be highly motivated to continue their musical pursuits, it might be relatively easy to obtain a volunteer musician from a local church or college to work with the individual. Local music teachers' groups also might provide a resource. The staff member could provide support in terms of setting up goals, objectives, practice schedules and space, and could also arrange for performing opportunities where appropriate. Residents with exceptional musical talent or ability could also be encouraged to take leadership roles in the facility's other music programs. One major difficulty often encountered with musically talented residents is their inability to accept a lower level of functioning. High levels of musical proficiency may have degenerated due to illness or lack of practice. Often, these individuals require much persuasion and support to help them realize that while they may not be able to achieve the degree of proficiency to which they may be accustomed, they can still participate in and be challenged by musical endeavors.

Recreational programming, both diversional and therapeutic, for nursing home residents who have special, individual needs can indeed present special challenges for activities professionals. Although this type of programming is usually more time-consuming than planning for large or small groups, the rewards are many. Structured time with residents can help build significant relationships, and provide the opportunity to monitor progress on a scale not often possible during group activities. It can promote self-esteem, because time is being set aside especially for a given person. It might also be helpful to enlist the assistance of social workers, physical therapists, nurses or volunteers to develop common goals and approaches to treatment. Activities professionals need to begin documenting what is being done in the area of individualized programming, and report results and observations to others in the field. By publishing and comparing enough case studies, it is hoped that patterns of response to various types of stimuli will emerge so that programming can become more systematic and more verifiable. Depending on the functioning levels of a given nursing home population, individualized activities may serve clients' needs better than group activities. Music offers many possibilities for meaningful interaction on an individualized basis. One resident at my facility summed up for me what can happen when quality time is set aside to meet an individualized need. After a music session, she smiled and said "You bring out the music in me."

CASE STUDY I

Miss A was admitted to the nursing facility in 1980 with a diagnosis of cardiovascular disease, increasing confusion and disorientation. Her personal hygiene had been neglected, and she began to require increased supervision for performance of activities of daily living (ADLs). She had also experienced several falls. Upon her admission, she could ambulate independently, and became involved in several group activities. As her overall health began to decline, her refusal to attend group activities increased. Due to a history of enjoyment of classical music and a background of both choir experience and piano study, she was included in the on-unit music therapy group. During group sessions, she demonstrated the ability to sing along on most songs, and to interact verbally with the therapist, or other group members if directed to do so. She attended the group for approximately 18 months, during which her social skills and cognitive abilities began to decline noticeably. She began dozing off during group sessions, and became unable to participate successfully within the group structure. She was also more frequently bed-bound. Individual music sessions were instituted approximately 18 months ago, and proved to be a positive alternative to group involvement. Miss A's verbalizations continued to evidence confused thought processes, and often consisted of gibberish plus one or two distinctive words. During individual sessions, Miss A responded to the music therapist with eye contact for approximately 80-90% of the 20 minute session. Her interest in the music was evidenced by a brightening of affect, and attempts to talk with the therapist. Eventually, two favorite hymns were identified with which Miss A could sing along. She was even able to tell the therapist when the keys were pitched too low. She began to comment favorably on songs, i.e., "that's good." The therapist noted some improvement in quality and content of verbalizations from the beginning to the end of the session, plus an increase in attention span as evidenced by Miss A's ability to attend to longer sessions. Miss A is now being reintegrated into the group setting.

CASE STUDY II

Mrs. B entered the nursing facility in 1984 with a diagnosis of chronic brain syndrome with dementia. She was admitted to the facility because of increased confusion causing inability to perform ADLs at the level required for residency in the domiciliary care facility where she had been living. She had a fall in 1985 and sustained a fracture of the left hip. This led to a decrease in independent mobility, and the patient began spending more time either in bed or confined to a geri-chair. She is frequently agitated, and verbalizes feelings of loneliness and the desire to go home. Shortly after admission, Mrs. B. expressed to the music therapist her interest and past involvement in music. For this reason, she was included in the on-unit music therapy group. She was able to participate in group tasks with minimal encouragement, up until the time of her fall in 1985. Following her hospitalization and return to the nursing home, a schedule of individual music visits was established, the goal of which was to decrease her level of agitation. Mrs. B. demonstrated a high level of anxiety prior to the hip fracture, and it is believed that the hospitalization and subsequent confinement increased this problem. When the music therapist would visit and find the patient anxious, the therapist would sing and play quiet hymns with a comforting theme on the autoharp. After a few minutes, Mrs. B. was able to focus her attention on the music, and even sing along on a few phrases. She particularly responded to "How Great Thou Art" which she could sing in its entirety in her native Swedish. She was able to verbalize about her loneliness and about missing her home. These feelings were validated by the therapist. She would comment on musical selections, and always thanked the therapist for the visit. During the session, relaxation of facial and arm muscles was noticed, along with a decrease in overall body movement. Often, Mrs. B. would fall asleep after the session.

REFERENCES

Bright, R. *Music in geriatric care*. Melville: Musicgraphics, 1980.
Feil, N. *V/F Validation The Feil Method How to help disoriented old-old*. Cleveland: Edward Feil Productions, 1982.
Foster, P. A multi-dimensional activities program. *Activities, Adaptation and Aging*, 1980, *1*(2), 35-39.
Gaston, E. *Music in therapy*. New York: Macmillan, 1968.

Appendix I

Sample Individual Music Session

Theme

Sports

Greeting Song:

"Oh What a Beautiful Mornin'"

Songs:

"Take Me Out to the Ballgame"

"Bicycle Built for Two"

"Row, Row, Row Your Boat"

Discussion:

Do you enjoy sports? Were you ever involved in sports? Do you have

a favorite ball team? Do you think that "life is but a dream?" Ask the

Appendix I, continued

resident to listen to the words of a given song, and ask questions about it.
For example, what kind of food is going to be bought in "Take Me Out to
the Ballgame?" (Peanuts and crackerjack)

Hymns:

Theme: "Sunshine"

"There is Sunshine in My Soul Today"
"Sun of My Soul"
"Brighten the Corner Where You Are"

Appendix II

INDIVIDUAL MUSIC VISITS - OBSERVATION REPORT

NAME _____

	DATES											COMMENTS
EYE COMMUNICATION												
Spontaneous eye contact												
Eye contact when directly addressed												
Approx. % eye contact during session												
Shut eyes												
Slept												
Easily distracted by outside noise												
FACIAL EXPRESSIONS												
Smiles, laughs												
Anxious appearance												
Depressed appearance												
Cries												
No discernible expression												
BODY LANGUAGE												
Movement in rhythm												
Spontaneous movement												
Rigid												
Reaches out toward sound source or therapist												
Perseveration of mvmt.												
VERBAL COMMUNICATION												
Verbalizes appropriately												
Attempts to verbalize												
Able to say "yes", "no"												
Non-verbal												
MUSICAL EXPRESSION												
Sings												
Hums melody of song												
Hums indiscernible melody												

Check all boxes where a response is observed.

Music Therapy and Hospice Care

Kristin G. Colligan

SUMMARY. The purpose of this article is to describe the hospice concept and to illustrate how music therapy activities can be incorporated into the concept. Included are suggestions for specific music activities plus supplementary activities which can be utilized with the aging patient. The final portion of this article is a set of case studies which very clearly indicate the validity of using music therapy with the terminally ill.

In recent years the philosophy towards care for the dying has changed dramatically. This holistic philosophy incorporates the whole person; body, mind, heart and soul. Prior to this current approach there was a distinct separation between physical and mental health. Physicians primarily treated the physical symptoms and psychotherapists treated the psychosocial aspects of health and well-being. Today it is extremely important to consider the workings of the mind and the body as interdependent parts of a whole system. In essence, we are working toward an integrated approach to health, which we will term the "holistic" healing process (Nowicki and Trevisan, 1978). The primary concern of the hospice is "good death." The primary goals of hospice are to control pain, ensure general comfort (both spiritual and mental), assure a dignified death for the patient, and give support and comfort to his family (Leone, 1980).

Music therapy can be effectively incorporated into the concept of palliative care. The role of music and music therapy is manifold. Not only can music serve as a comfort emotionally and

Kristin G. Colligan, RMT, is the Music Therapist at Powhatan Nursing Home, Falls Church, Virginia. Kristin completed her internship at Forbes Health System, Pittsburgh, PA, at which time she gained her hospice experience.

spiritually and as a "time passer" during a period of fear but also as an outlet for feelings of anger and aggression, and a diversion from pain; and it promotes relaxation which in turn can raise the threshold of pain.

Music therapy activities provide worthwhile and meaningful activities which can alleviate the inactivity and self-pity which comes at the "time of dying." Music therapy can also help to ease the sense of isolation that often comes with an advanced illness. Many patients will withdraw from their painful reality. In order to help the patient, activities should consider the following as cited in the Occupational Therapy Newsletter, April, 1976.

1. Activities should be short-term and reality oriented.
2. This may be the first time the patient has "time on his hands" and the therapist can help him learn a craft, skill, become involved in music, painting, poetry and recreational activities at his ability and tolerance levels.
3. The patient may pick up and carry on a hobby he has enjoyed in the past.
4. Hobbies and activities can serve as a reality maintenance.

The terminally ill patient faces a time of regression and dependency as the disease becomes more advanced. The patient may become increasingly more depressed as he loses more ability to function. Music therapy can be used to rebuild self-esteem and self-image.

Also cited in the Occupational Therapy Newsletter, 1976 are the following points on the value of music therapy.

1. The therapist can help the patient retain his sense of identity and individuality by becoming involved in a skill or activity that will foster creativity and produce something that will provide the needed gratification and increase the self-image.
2. The therapist can help focus on the patient's remaining capabilities and help maintain his maximum functioning (physically).
3. The therapist can provide spiritual music which would add to his support during this time.

Anxiety and the fear of dying often produce tension and the loss of self-control. The therapist can help to restore a measure of this self-control by creating a structured environment, and yet one that fosters open communication and the freedom to share personal feelings. The knowledge and availability plus the sympathetic understanding of the therapist can contribute immeasurably to the patient's adjustment to his problem during this period of stress when everything in his environment seems to be conspiring against him (American Cancer Society, 1963). The Occupational Therapy Newsletter, 1976, describes how the therapist can create an accepting environment.

1. The therapist can provide support by allowing the patient to talk about his feelings about dying. By talking it over he feels less rejected and abandoned.
2. How a person feels about his dying is affected by those around him; his family and the professional staff involved in his care. The family and staff should be educated and helped to understand what the patient is experiencing, physically and emotionally.
3. The therapist can help the family by letting them know the patient's attitude and feelings so that visits can be meaningful and pleasant.

The therapist also helps patients become involved socially and involved in activities that provide a sense of normalcy. The therapist can aid the patient in increasing his living space, as the dying tend to limit it through withdrawal, isolation and disinterest (Occupational Therapy Newsletter, 1978). The therapist considers all facets of his client. Because music has a number of facets as well, and a number of capabilities that contribute to its psychotherapeutic use, it opens avenues of verbal and nonverbal communication that has been called the language of the emotions (Nowicki and Trevisan, 1978). These avenues of communication are stressed within the hospice. Therefore music can be successfully incorporated into a hospice setting.

A hospice is a unique facility which is designed to care for the terminally ill. The Oxford English Dictionary defines a hospice as a house of rest and entertainment for pilgrims, travellers or strangers . . . for the destitute or the sick. The following are the governmentally defined regulations of hospice care: a program which provides palliative and supportive care for terminally ill patients and their families, either directly or on a consulting basis with the patient's physician, an organized program of care and care extends through the mourning process. Emphasis is placed on symptom control and preparation before and after death (Stoddard, 1978).

The hospice is a caring community which promotes physical, emotional and spiritual well-being. There are highly trained professionals on the staff plus numerous helpers which include volunteers and family members. It has its own set of values and is autonomous in terms of professional procedure.

The philosophy of a typical hospice with inpatient services incorporate all these ideas plus several other important aspects: to provide the patient with the freedom to make personal choices regarding his or her care; to alleviate loneliness and anxiety through fostering open communication between patient and family; to create awareness among patient's family; health care providers and the public concerning the needs of the dying (Forbes Hospice Pamphlet, 1980). Inpatient services are usually provided in a small unit designed to permit unrestricted visiting so that patients, family members, friends, and even family pets spend as much time together as possible. In addition to the patient's private rooms, often there is a communal dining room and kitchen, where patients and family can prepare their own meals and snacks if desired. Usually the aim of an inpatient stay is to prepare the patient and family for a return to home care. However, certain physical needs arise that may preclude a patient's return home.

Through the hospice home care component, all services provided in the inpatient unit can be extended to those patients who choose to return, or remain from the onset, at home with a responsible caregiver. Bereavement support is also offered to families in this program, as well as others who may wish to avail themselves of it. The same interdisciplinary team serves inpatient, home care, and bereavement components.

Patient and family meet with the hospice team in order to evaluate medical and social needs, review services offered, including spiritual support and develop a plan of care. Clergy of the family's choice, as well as any other consultation that is requested are invited to participate in care.

An individual who is facing an imminent death has many needs which include psychosocial, physical, social, leisure and spiritual. The psychosocial needs are best defined by Dr. Elizabeth Kübler-Ross. She has categorized these feelings into five stages. The five stages are denial, anger, bargaining, depression, and acceptance. It must be made clear that a patient will experience these feelings in different orders sometimes, and may go back to one stage or another. The first stage is denial. Denial functions as a buffer after unexpected shocking news, allows the patient to collect himself and with time mobilize other defenses (Fordice, 1972). This initial time for the patient is very difficult. He is being bombarded by doctors, family, financial burdens, fear of isolation and disfigurement. It is only natural that the patient would escape through means of denial of some sort.

The stage after denial is anger. This includes rage, envy, and resentment. It is logical for the patient to ask "WHY ME?." Feelings of anger are difficult to cope with, not only for the family of the patient but also the staff. Anger is displaced in all directions and projected on the environment at times almost at random (Kübler-Ross, 1969). Nothing seems to satisfy the patient. Frustration and anxiety run very high for staff, family and patient. Staff must be very considerate and allow the person this time. The client will soon lessen his demands once most of the anger is released. A patient who is respected and understood, who is given attention and a little time, will soon lower his voice and reduce his angry demands. He will know that he is a valuable human being, cared for, allowed to function at the highest level as long as he can (Kübler-Ross, 1969).

This patient will be listened to without the need to raise his voice for attention and the staff will be more understanding. They will make more visits to the patient which will increase the positive attitudes of the patient. He will begin to feel more important and valuable. The attitudes of the staff and family are crucial to the patient's well-being.

As the patient's attitudes improve and sense of identity is restored he may begin to bargain for time. The third stage is bargaining. Kübler-Ross theorizes that bargaining is really an attempt to postpone; it has to include a prize offered "for good behavior," it also sets a self-imposed "deadline" . . . and it includes an implicit promise that the patient will not ask for more if this one postponement is granted.

Sometimes these promises are a result of feelings of guilt. Perhaps the patient feels he owes something in life or he feels he owes someone something for a past favor. It is the therapist's responsibility to help the patient discover the depth and reasons for his feeling. This period usually does not last long for the patient soon realizes that the bargains are not going to be fulfilled or if they are, he really isn't getting any more time.

This bargaining period precedes the fourth stage of depression. The terminally ill patient can no longer deny his illness and faces many burdens as well as many losses. The patient finally begins to prepare himself for the impending death. It seems that he too must go through a period of grief for his own death. Kübler-Ross differentiates between two types of depression: reactive and preparatory. Each must be treated in a special way.

The cause of the reactive depression is easily identified and alleviated by easing some of the unrealistic guilt and shame. Building self-esteem and giving recognition helps the patient function in the role of which he is still capable. The depression lifts when vital issues are taken care of.

The second type of depression is the result of impending loss rather than past loss. The first reaction to this behavior is to try to cheer the patient. At this point, it is probably better to help the patient face his feelings in the sorrow. The client needs to cope with these feelings in order to bring him closer to acceptance. The therapist acts as a facilitator who aids the patient in expression of the feelings. Kübler-Ross believes that families should know that this type of depression is necessary and beneficial if the patient is to die in a stage of acceptance and peace.

The final stage is that of acceptance. This stage is reached when the patient has been given some help in working through the previously described stages. He will no longer be depressed nor angry and he will be beyond mourning for impending loss. He will enter a stage of quiet expectancy. The patient will also sleep a lot. This should not be taken as a sign of resignation but a sign of acceptance and preparation. Communication often becomes more nonverbal than verbal.

Visits from the therapist take on a new form, becoming very simple. Few words may be spoken and only meaningful gestures used. Some moments of silence may be the most meaningful communications for people who are not uncomfortable in the presence of a dying person. The therapist's presence may be all the assurance the patient needs — he knows he won't be alone.

Throughout all these stages the patient still has some other needs must be met. Many physical needs must be cared for, and of primary concern to the patient is relief and diversion from pain. Sometimes the pain is so great that the patient ceases to be aware of what is going on around him. If this is the case, how can the patient possibly cope with the emotions he is feeling also. The purpose of proper pain control is to help the patient die with dignity and humility and without strain and aching. A primary factor, of concern to physicians and nurses caring for dying patients, is the amount of pain an individual has; it is very difficult to maintain emotional equilibrium when you are in extreme pain (Kübler-Ross, 1975). If the patient feels he is in control of his pain then he can also control his routines including his emotions and feelings about his impending death. A patient will have a greater peace if he knows that his suffering will be kept at a bearable minimum. Thus, relaxation contributes greatly to the peace of a dying patient. The patient may feel an increased amount of body tension and rigidity as the result of stress, anxiety, and pain. The patient needs to relax for many reasons but one of the most important reasons is to break the pain cycle. That is, when the pain begins, greater pain is anticipated, therefore causing anxiety which in turn causes the patient to experience more pain. This vicious cycle can be interrupted by utilizing relaxation techniques. The therapist uses relaxation techniques with music, guided imagery, and diversion so that the patient's attention is not self-directed. In addition an environment which induces relaxation can be created. The therapist can also help the patient conceptualize the pain by supplying the means by which the patient can describe his pain (an abstract feeling) in concrete terms.

Oftentimes the pain and disfigurement of terminal illness can cause a patient to isolate himself. He loses opportunities for socialization and cuts ties with the community. This self-induced isolation prevents the patient from sharing with others who might be facing similar situations. The feelings of isolation may also be caused by family or friends who are unable to accept the patient's illness and death. These individuals do not visit or communicate, leaving the patient very much alone.

Another area to consider regarding a patient who is receiving palliative care is his ongoing need for leisure and recreational pursuits. Although the patient may be unable to actively participate in hobbies or activities he can still be involved in passive or vicarious endeavors. The patient can observe a live musical performance or theatrical production. Although he is not on stage, he can relive the performance in his mind. The introduction of music therapy can provide the opportunity to learn a new hobby or revive an interest in music.

Finally, one of the last and probably most critical needs of the dying patient is that of his spiritual nature. An individual must come to terms with life and death. These matters will involve not only family relationships but also the relationship to God and belief in heaven or hell. Seldom is there an individual who doesn't wrestle with these questions even if he has been a professed atheist. The patient's move through a transition of struggle and anxiety to receptivity and tranquility as he or she yields to the "unseen divine." This resolution parallels the stage of acceptance.

DESIGNING MUSIC THERAPY ACTIVITIES TO MEET THE NEEDS OF THE HOSPICE PATIENT

The presentation of music as therapy to an individual who is terminally ill can be very delicate. It is important to introduce music therapy in a manner that highlights the universality of music. The therapist must be well informed on the patient's background and nature of illness. With this knowledge, communication between therapist and patient is facilitated. Sometimes using a music preference inventory with sample pieces is a simple way to break the ice.

In the use of music therapy with the terminally ill and those dealing with the death of a loved one, many therapeutic techniques can be incorporated into the treatment plan. Instrumental music listening and improvisational music therapy with the client playing an instrument to reflect the inner state, may serve to elicit the release of limbic tensions (Nowicki and Trevisan, 1978). The limbic system functions to produce such emotional feelings as fear, anger, pleasure, and sorrow, which in turn can modify the way a person acts. More specifically, the limbic system seems to recognize imbalances in a person's physical or psychological condition that might threaten survival. By causing pleasant or unpleasant feelings about experiences, the limbic system guides the person into behavior that is likely to ensure survival.

Before the feelings of pleasure elicited by the limbic system can be released, the patient must be willing and have actively chosen music therapy to help in his preparation for death. The music therapist helps the patient with facing reality during the period of denial and isolation. The therapist represents reality and because he is a member of the staff, his visits prevent the patient from being isolated or from isolating himself. Others withdraw from the patient—family and friends. This withdrawal is often the result of confused feelings about the illness. Communication by a variety of not so subtle behaviors indicates that the patient is already viewed as part of the unknown world of the hereafter by those around him. This leaves the patient feeling isolated.

The person with cancer must assume the additional burden of a most difficult role. The patient too often must become the initiator of a therapeutic and sustaining relationship in his efforts to be an active participant in life (Bouchard and Owens, 1972). The music therapist provides opportunities for the patient to talk, although conversation may be superficial. As rapport and trust develops between client and therapist through honesty and sincerity, the music therapist can bring in background music which may act as a facilitator for conversation as well as fill in the uncomfortable silences that can evolve at this time.

Soft, melodic, lightly orchestrated non-percussive music is the most appropriate type to use in this situation. Although the patient may be unaware of the benefits of this music, it stimulates the limbic system. When the appropriate music is used it can elicit pleasant sensations from the limbic system. It is important to find the music that best suits the client because some music may be stimulative and some sedative.

Sedative music is of a sustained melodic nature, with strong rhythmic and percussive elements largely lacking. This results in physical sedation and responses of an intellectual and contemplative nature rather than physical (Gaston, 1968).

Music that is pre-categorized as sedative is not always relaxing, this depends upon the individual listener. The therapist with the cooperation of the patient, must determine what type of music is sedative. In the case studies to follow, you will find that Vivaldi's "Four Seasons" is relaxing to one, while Grofe's "Grand Canyon Suite" is relaxing to another. Using background music is a simple way to ease the patient into a state of passive listening. The patient need not interact but listens to the music and allows it to minister in any way that the patient wills it. Passive listening allows for reflection and contemplation. The aim of the music is to help listeners develop self-awareness, clarify personal values, release blocked-up psychic energy sources, enrich group spirit, bring about deep relaxation, and foster religious experience (Bonny and Savary, 1973).

This deep awareness helps the patient identify specific feelings. If the patient is in the anger stage and has identified these feelings then specific music selections and activities can be provided. Rhythmic music, coupled with movement, playing percussive instruments to strong rhythms, e.g., tambourine, can aid in the release of anger (Nowicki and Trevisan, 1978). Musical preference is also an indicator of feelings. Choices of music can present a passive catharsis of feelings rather than an active — playing how you feel. As with H.Q., a hospice patient and music therapy client, who asked for loud percussive classical pieces. She was experiencing a lot of anger, especially at God and her family. She was able to express this anger in an appropriate and acceptable manner.

After the anger period comes the bargaining stage. It is difficult to pinpoint specific music therapy activities to use at this time, other than to provide music as an emotional outlet and familiar mode of comfort. However, consistency of treatment as well as patient support by the therapist is most important throughout the entire period of the dying process.

Emotional support is especially crucial through the depression period. It is essential therefore to provide a variety of activities that keep the patient too busy to become preoccupied with himself. Providing activities that allow the patient to function at his fullest capacity are the best in this case. Some activities used with a patient who vacillated between depression and acceptance include: writing poetry to music — using music as the stimulus for thought processes and for the theme, reading selections from poetry, prose and the Bible, creating collages using background music as the theme for the pictures, creating a story using music and appropriate pictures and singing special songs including hymns.

The hymns and scripture reading are very important factors at this time as the patient nears his death. The patient is attempting to sort out his spiritual self from his worldly self. For many years the Bible has offered much comfort and now the need for it is crucial. Relaxing music combined with scriptures: the Psalms, the Beatitudes, selections from the books of Paul and also from Revelation give the patient a sense of his spiritual self, that which will perpetuate after his death. For example:

> And there are heavenly bodies and earthly bodies; the beauty that belongs to heavenly bodies is different from the beauty that belongs to earthly bodies. The sun has its own beauty, the moon another beauty, and the stars a different beauty; and even among the stars there are different kinds of beauty. (Good News Bible, 1976)

By contemplating these thoughts and feelings and allowing them to become integrated into his thought process, the patient can gain great insights about himself.

The individual learns that even in death there is beauty. Although he may be disfigured or handicapped in some way, the dying patient retains dignity and humility in the knowledge that he is still an important person. This is the main goal of music therapy in the hospice — a person is still a worthwhile and sensitive individual who still has a place in the hearts of man and God.

This reassurance is reinforced by music therapy. This assurance gives the patient faith, hope and love. The greatest of these is love (Good News Bible, 1976).

> I may be able to speak the languages of men and even of angels, but if I have no love, my speech is no more than a noisy gong or a clanging bell. I may have the gift of inspired preaching; I may have all knowledge and understand all secrets; I may have all the faith to move mountains — but if I have no love, I am nothing, I may give away everything I have, and even give up my body to be burned — but if I have no love, this does me no good. (Good News Bible, 1976)

The therapist shows love in all actions in dealing with dying patients. It is most evident during the patient's journey to acceptance. The patient might just want the therapist to hold his hand. This has been a long journey and client and therapist have shared it. The needs of the dying grow fewer as the days increase.

M.P., a hospice patient, desired only hymns, scripture reading and the Lord's Prayer towards the last few days. M.P. had specific needs and was able to define them and design her own treatment plan. She knew what help she needed in order to reach the final acceptance of love — God's love. I must stress again that each patient has individual needs throughout this last journey of the worldly life.

Pain is a common fact through the journey of almost every terminally ill patient. It is felt as a specific sensation with its intensity determined by the extent of tissue damage. This theory views pain as a simple transmission from the source of stimulation (nerve receptors) directly to specific pain-center location within the brain (Wolfe, 1978).

In the hospice, the staff and the patient work together to reduce the pain. The patient knows his pain threshold and knows when the medicine is necessary. Therefore, he can ask for it when he needs it. There are other methods to ease pain. Encouraging deep relaxation is one method. The music therapist can choose music and activities which can induce this deep level of relaxation. Helen L. Bonny, founder of the Institute for Consciousness and Music and research music therapist at the Maryland Psychiatric

Research Center, has devised a method of relaxation using contingent music. The goal of feeling relaxed is feeling weightless. Feeling weightless means that the body's muscles are in equilibrium or balance. When the muscles of the entire body are in this state of balance or weightlessness, the body is totally relaxed. This sensation of relaxation would help any dying patient have a better sense of well-being.

In order to achieve this deep relaxation, one must begin by making the patient as physically comfortable as possible. To relax, an individual must consciously suggest his body to relax. Then follow this recommended procedure: begin by fixing the mind on the feet and relax them — this may be done by flexing the muscles if possible then relaxing them, then the legs, the arms, abdomen, chest, throat, facial muscles, and eyes. Another technique is to suggest a light source, the sun, or a sunlamp which is focusing warmth and energy to each body part which in turn suggests comfort and relaxation. Each in turn should yield to suggestion until complete relaxation is achieved. Breath flow is also important and it should be steady, regular and smooth. Relaxation should take place before the listening experience begins.

The mind can be directed to concentrate when the body is relaxed. The attention is now focused. The patient is able to focus attention on the next procedure called induction. Begin by having the patient visualize a doorway; he opens the door to see soft twilight mist. A long winding staircase can be seen as the patient moves from one step to the next, count down slowly from ten to zero. When the patient reaches zero, he senses a change, his feet are firmly on the ground and the mist has cleared. The patient has now entered a new level of consciousness and is ready to let the music take him wherever he wants to go (Bonny and Savary, 1973).

The therapist guides the patient through an individual journey. The therapist facilitates this relaxation process. Once the procedure is firmly established in the patient's mind, he can do the relaxation process independently. It is still important; however, for the therapist to choose the music. Even more vital is the discussion that ensues after the listening portion of the exercise. The discussion opens up many avenues and insights about the patient and his feelings, and needs to be guided by a therapist. Not only is this activity valuable in aiding relaxation, but also in redirecting the patient's thoughts of himself to others. Memories, colors, shapes emotions can all be elicited through this music therapy technique. Combining spiritual readings with this altered state of consciousness can help the patient also come to terms with his spiritual identify. Other activities and music selections using this deep relaxation technique can be found in Helen L. Bonny and Louis Savary's book, *Music and Your Mind*. Music can be a nonverbal expression of the many emotions that a dying patient experiences.

The following descriptions are more than just case studies. These are true to life experiences shared between patient and therapist. A beautiful rapport developed between patient and therapist. Sharing of all moments became very important. Perhaps the intensity of the relationship is not realized until after the patient dies.

I must stress that each patient is an individual with very specific needs. The therapist must be emotionally and spiritually prepared as well as have the therapeutic background and counseling skills necessary to work with the terminally ill. Music is a powerful medium, and a person is defenseless against its impact on the emotions. The terminally ill person already faces much emotional upheaval. Music can comfort, reach and bring pleasure, but it may also touch hidden pains, memories and suffering which will have to be worked through and possibly resolved to assure healing of a person's inner being. The therapist must be able to facilitate such a process and integrate its outcome into the general treatment plan of the patient (Munro, 1984). The following will illustrate a small portion of the many ways in which a therapist is needed.

CASE STUDY I

M.P. was an 82-year-old woman diagnosed with terminal cancer. The cancer began abdominally and metastasized throughout her body. The patient had taught piano lessons for many years. Her interest level in music was very high. Also, M.P. was Catholic and found great comfort in the Lord throughout her lifetime.

Since the patient had a prior interest in piano music, beginning treatments were directed towards this interest. Recordings of piano music and live performances of familiar pieces were used to help the therapist establish a therapeutic relationship with the patient. M.P. liked a variety of music, including recordings of the classics, and familiar sing-a-long tunes. She found these activities very enjoyable and always told the therapist what she liked and didn't like.

As the therapist discovered what type of music to which the patient had the greatest positive response, the therapist was able to incorporate the pieces into relaxation exercises. In order to facilitate relaxation, music was first listened to and while the selection continued, scripture and prayers were included. The patient had always found great comfort and pleasure in the words of the Bible, especially the 23rd Psalm. Therefore, this passage was used quite frequently. The music that coincided with the reading was quiet and soothing. The patient took upon a passive listening role, allowing the music and verse to minister. M.P. always responded positively and often expressed: "you have no idea how much better I feel." Music therapy was usually held after the patient had gone back to bed. The procedure of getting to bed from chair was very painful for her so she needed music therapy to help her relax and divert her mind from the immediate and ensuing pain. Overt signs of relaxation could be noted in M.P.'s face and body. No longer was there a furrowed brow and there was less rigidity in her body.

As M.P. came nearer to death she desired fewer things from the music therapist in terms of activities but she still needed the support and the presence the therapist offered. M.P. liked each session to follow a pattern: the treatment began with two hymns, then the Scripture reading followed by the Lord's Prayer and the treatment itself usually ended with M.P.'s favorite hymn, "In the Garden." M.P. liked the therapist to remain with her awhile and perhaps just hold her hand or play the piano softly — songs that had special meaning to her. The therapist provided great comfort during M.P.'s last few days. Shortly before M.P. died, she said to the therapist: "Thank-you so much, I never could have done it without you. God really loves us." M.P. reached her ultimate understanding, she had searched for the answer to her question: "Does God love me?" M.P. found it, and attained her acceptance. Music therapy had helped her in her journey.

CASE STUDY II

G.R. was a 68-year-old man whose cancer began in his prostate gland and metastasized throughout the lower portion of his body. When this client entered the hospice he was very tense, anxious and talkative. G.R.'s body appeared very tense and he frequently asked for pain medication. G.R. also talked continuously. This seemed to indicate an anxiety which he was not revealing to staff or to the music therapist. It appeared that this patient was attempting to conceal or ignore certain conditions that might have been bothering him.

The patient made many requests for specific music selections. The therapist had to do research in order to satisfy his desire and need. Often when the music selection was played, G.R. talked through most of the piece, occasionally the topic of conversation coincided with the theme of the music. It was the therapist's responsibility to interpret and sift through this stream of conversation. It seemed that the patient could have been behaving in this way to conceal feelings or to just relate personal experiences and not feelings, or possibly he felt the need to entertain the therapist. It also may have been an acceptable and appropriate way for G.R. to release anxiety, nervousness, and tension. The therapist designed activities which directed this energy into creative expression. These activities compensated for the energy usually spent talking.

The activities began with passive listening. By playing guitar and singing for G.R., the therapist was able to interrupt the conversational pattern by giving G.R. the role of an audience. This activity facilitated relaxation by allowing the patient to take a passive role. The music acted primarily as a diversion from pain at this point. Music and relaxation were utilized later to ease pain. As the pattern for listening was established, the therapist was then able to slowly introduce a new type of listening—active listening. Choosing appropriate pieces from G.R.'s requests and then using guided discussion, the therapist was able to control topics of discussion. These topics were viewed in much greater depth, which allowed not only the therapist to gain greater insight about the patient, but also the patient gained greater knowledge of himself.

When this insightful discussion begun, the therapist could implement other activities such as: writing poetry to music. Program music, which has a theme, is the best way to establish a mood. Stories can also be written this way, using music to set the theme. Creating original compositions through improvisation can also be beneficial. Putting together collages and drawing which illustrates how the music makes you feel are also valuable activities. Not only is it a creative effort completed by the patient but also a visual reinforcer that the patient is still capable of more. These activities may seem only diversionary but they are actually much more. Creating original works provides the reinforcement of self-esteem. Although a patient may be physically disabled he is still of value to those around him.

As G.R.'s treatment continued, he grew weaker. Topics were discussed in much greater depth, and superficial conversation was minimal. Even the topics G.R. chose were very significant in approaching the stage of acceptance. G.R. talked openly about funerals, he talked about love and the role it played in his life. G.R. began to request the therapist to read selections with spiritual overtones, with background music. After one such treatment, G.R. said: "Boy that music, and those words sure do paint pictures in my mind." G.R. then proceeded to vividly describe these pictures. G.R. seemed to be searching at this time. Sometimes it is difficult for the therapist to identify the searching but he can act as the facilitator. The therapist asked G.R. how he believed music therapy had helped him during this time. G.R. replied: "The music took my mind off myself and put it on important matters, otherwise I would have been worrying about my illness. Besides, I love music and I can express myself." At the end of another treatment session G.R. said: "You know, I can't tell anyone else but you (referring to the therapist) how I feel. Everyone else would say I was crazy. But with you I can tell how the music and the words really make me feel with all the flowery words that I want to use. I can really tell you how I feel." Once again music therapy appropriately directed the dying patient through the five stages of death.

CASE STUDY III

H.Q. was a 64-year-old woman. When H.Q. entered the hospice she had recently had a colostomy. She would have nothing to do with the colostomy care or acknowledge that it was a part of her daily routine. H.Q. talked constantly of her two brothers and her boss. She expressed many mixed emotions towards them. At times she was angry, other times she said she was very guilty about how she treated them. H.Q. also had many "conversations with God," asking for more time and less time. She said that if she had more time she could make up everything to her brothers for being a burden to them. It was obvious to the therapist and those associated with H.Q., that she needed help in alleviating the guilt and resolving the anger she felt. H.Q. enjoyed coming into the lounge and listening to the therapist play the piano and sing. H.Q. made a variety of requests depending on the mood she was in. Sometimes songs were reminiscent of days gone by and other times the selections indicated anger or melancholy. On days she verbally expressed anger, H.Q. requested loud percussive pieces, on days that she expressed sadness and loss H.Q. requested smooth melodic pieces by Chopin and Mozart. H.Q. preferred live music over the recordings. She said: "You can listen to music on the radio or record player any day but there won't be many more days when I can hear a live performance." H.Q. usually initiated the topic of discussion. The therapist's role was primarily that of a listener and sounding board. H.Q. made it very clear to the therapist that only she would make judgements on what she was saying and that she only wanted the therapist to listen.

H.Q. was a most challenging patient because each day she was experiencing a different step in her journey toward acceptance. The therapist had to be very patient and be prepared for whatever H.Q. needed to say. Towards the last days, H.Q. slipped gently into a quiet stage of acceptance. The only music she desired was live piano music. H.Q.'s needs became centralized and defined, the therapist simply fulfilled one of her few last wishes.

CONCLUSION

Few welcome death as a preferable alternative to the beauty and challenge of life. While dying is the inevitable and final act of living, most individuals concentrate their thoughts on the quality of living even to the moment of departure. It is therefore essential that the integrated efforts of the support team be directed towards enrichment of the patient's remaining life, and, at the same time assist family, friends, trusted professional attendants, and clergy to the patient's need for contemplation of the circumstances of death (Kübler-Ross, 1969). Music can add beauty and the composition of music can add the challenge. Although death is a final act, music can illustrate the immortality of the dying patient, either by the patient's original composition or by hearing those of others. This reinforces the patient's spiritual self-concept. Music helps add dimension and quality by expanding the awareness of the world and those in it. Music can enrich the life of the patient and also add to the good memories that the family has of that patient. Words and music open avenues for the patient to explore his mind and soul. He may know he is dying but he will also be assured that he is still a beautiful and unique person.

> The angel also showed me the river of the water of life, sparkling like crystal, and coming from the throne of God and the Lamb and flowing down the middle of the city's street. On each side of the river was the tree of life, which bears fruit twelve times a year, once each month; and its leaves are for healing the nations. (Good News Bible, 1976)

The patient will bear fruit many times before he dies. The words he speaks will be like a flowing river, endlessly sharing the wisdom he has found in this worldly life. He will search for the wisdom to be found in his eternal life. When this search is over, the words which flow from his mouth will be songs of thanks and gratefulness.

REFERENCES

A Cancer Sourcebook for Nurses, American Cancer Society, 1963.

Bourchard, Rosemary and Norma Owens, *Nursing Care of the Cancer Patient*, C. V. Mosby Company, St. Louis, 1972.

Fordice, Janice, *"Communicating with the Dying Patient,"* summarized from *On Death and Dying*, Elizabeth Kübler-Ross and *Awareness of Dying*, Barney Blazer, Minneapolis VA Hospital, January 27, 1972.

Gaston, E. Thayer, *Music in Therapy*, McMillan Publishing Co., Inc., New York, 1968.

Hole, John W., *Human Anatomy and Physiology*, Wm. C. Brown Company Publishers, Dubuque, Iowa, 1978.

Kübler-Ross, Elizabeth, *Death: The Final Stage of Growth*, Prentice-Hall, Inc., New Jersey, 1975.

———, *On Death and Dying*, McMillan Publishing Co., New York, 1969.

Leone, Louis A., "The Concept of Hospice," *Oncology Times*, September 1980, Vol. II, no. 9.

Munro, Susan, *Music Therapy in Palliative/Hospice Care*, Magnamusic-Baton, St. Louis, Missouri, 1984.

Nowicke, Alicia and Lonnie Trevisan, *Beyond the Sound: A Technical and Philosophical Approach to Music Therapy*, U.S.A., 1978.

Occupational Therapy Newsletter, April 1976, Volume 30, no. 4. Death and Dying Seminar at Fairfield Hills Hospital, Newton Connecticut, Frances Teicholz OTR.

Stoddard, Sandol, *The Hospice Movement: A Better Way of Caring for the Dying*, Vintage Books, New York, 1978.

Taylor, Dale B., "Subject Responses to Precategorized Stimulative and Sedative Music," *Journal of Music Therapy*, Vol. X, Summer 1973, pp. 86-84.

Wolfe, David E. "Pain Rehabilitation and Music Therapy," *Journal of Music Therapy*, Vol. XV (4), 1978, pp. 162-176.

Music as Sleep Therapy

The therapeutic value of music is great for easing one into a night of beautiful, healing sleep. After you have completed your bedtime ritual of prayers, readings—whatever is your custom—try singing yourself to sleep without ever emitting a sound.

I can not sing! I can not carry a tune! But in my mind's ear I sing with perfect pitch, lilting trills and lovely glissando modulations. With body relaxed and weary from physical exercise, I concentrate completely on singing three stanzas of "Holy, Holy, Holy" followed by three stanzas of "Come, Thou Almighty King." Sleep usually comes before the end of the third stanza.

For those who prefer patriotic or secular songs to religious ones, suggestions are: "My Country 'Tis of Thee," "In the Shade of the Old Apple Tree," and "Ah, Sweet Mystery of Life," one line of which: "All the longing, striving, waiting, yearning, and the burning hopes, the joy and idle tears that fall!" is especially effective for letting go of the care of the day and sinking into the arms of Morpheus.

The choice of songs is of course an individual matter but the memorizing of the music stanzas of the songs chosen is absolutely necessary as is the complete concentration on the singing.

Vida Hickerson
Age 88

Resource List

Compiled by Michael Lewallen

SONG ANTHOLOGIES

75 SONGS 1890-1920
World Library Series
The Big 3 Music Corporation
New York, NY

A good collection, available in music stores. Recommended.

THOSE WONDERFUL
  YEARS – 89
UNFORGETTABLE
SONGS FROM 1920-1940
Compiled and edited by
Dick Stern
The Big 3 Music Corporation
New York, NY

Recommended.

Reader's Digest Series
  FAMILY SONGBOOK
  POPULAR SONGS
    THAT WILL
    LIVE FOREVER
  FESTIVAL OF
    POPULAR SONGS
  TREASURY OF BEST-
    LOVED SONGS
  MERRY CHRISTMAS
    SONGBOOK
  FAMILY SONGBOOK
    OF FAITH AND JOY

Wide variety of songs, sturdy bindings. Recommended. Available from Reader's Digest, Inc., or at bookstores and music stores.

UNFORGETTABLE
MUSICAL
MEMORIES
REMEMBERING
 YESTERDAY'S HITS
COUNTRY AND WEST-
ERN SONGBOOK

BEST-LOVED SONGS
 OF THE
 AMERICAN PEOPLE
Ed. Denes Agay
Doubleday & Company, Inc.
Garden City, NY

Available hard-bound or with spiral binding — recommended. Songs arranged chronologically.

BERLIN'S BEST SONG
 FOLIO, VOL 1
Irving Berlin Music
Corp.
1290 Avenue of the Americas
New York, NY 10104

Available at music stores. Most Berlin songs are available only from this publisher.

Fake Books
(There are many good ones.)

Fake Books usually contain several hundred songs, with melodies, lyrics, and chords only.

BEST SONGS OF THE 20s
 AND 30s
Great Songs of the Century
 Series
Warner Brothers
Publications, Inc.
75 Rockefeller Plaza
New York, NY 10019

TAKE ME OUT TO THE
 BALLGAME
 AND OTHER FAVORITE
 SONG HITS OF 1906-
 1908

Ed. Lester Levy
Dover Publications, Inc.
NY

THEY DON'T WRITE
  SONGS LIKE THESE
  ANYMORE, VOL. II
Amsco Music Publishing Co.
Division of Music
Sales Corp.
33 W. 60th St.
New York, NY 10023

SING ALONG SENIOR   Has large-type lyrics.
  CITIZENS
Comp. Roy E. Grant
Charles C. Thomas,
  Publisher
301-327 E. Lawrence Ave.
Springfield, IL 62717

SONG HITS OF THE
  ROARING TWENTIES
Warner Brothers
Publications, Inc.
75 Rockefeller Plaza
New York, NY 10019

WORLD'S GREATEST
  HITS OF THE SWING
  ERA FROM 1920-1939
Comp. and ed.
Jim Armstrong
Hansen House
1870 West Ave.
Miami Beach, FL 33139A

TRIBUTE TO AMERICA
Creative Concepts
Publishing Corp.
Distributed by Lewis Music

Publishing Corp.
263 Veterans Blvd.
Carlstadt, NJ 07072

THE NEW BLUE BOOK OF FAVORITE SONGS Schmitt, Hall & McCreary Minneapolis, MN	Includes "The Golden Book of Favorite Songs" and "The Gray Book of Favorite Songs," plus supplements.
PARADOLOGY: SONGS FOR FUN AND FELLOWSHIP Author E. O. Harbin Cokesbury Press Nashville, TN	Copyright 1927, out of print. Contains dozens of fun songs which the author has written using popular tunes. An excellent source for greeting songs. Might be found in used book shops or church libraries.

MUSICAL EQUIPMENT COMPANIES

Rhythm Band, Inc.
P.O. Box 126
Fort Worth, TX 76101

Sound Education
263 Huntington Avenue
Boston, MA 02115
(617) 266-4727,
(617) 266-8165

Suzuki Musical
Instrument Corp.
P.O. Box 261030
San Diego, CA 92126

SOURCES FOR BOOKS AND OTHER MATERIALS

MMB Music, Inc.
10370 Page Industrial Blvd.
Saint Louis, MO 63132
(314) 427-5660

Many books and resource
materials in Music Therapy
and related fields. Catalog
available.

Potentials Development
775 Main Street
Buffalo, NY 14203

BOOKS, VARIOUS TOPICS

*The American Heritage of the
20's and 30's*
American Heritage Publishing Co., Inc.
NY, 1970.

Bonny, Helen L., and
Savary, Louis M.
Music and Your Mind
Collins Associates
 Publishing, Inc.
Harper and Row, Publishers
NY, 1973.

Contains information about
Guided Imagery with Music.

Bright, Ruth.
Music in Geriatric Care.
Musicgraphics,
Belwin-Mills
 Publishing Corp.
Melville, NY, 1980.

Bright, Ruth.
*Practical Planning in
 Music Therapy
 for the Aged.*
Musicgraphics,
Belwin-Mills

Publishing Corp.
Melville, NY

Brooks, Elston.
I've Heard Those Songs
  Before: The Weekly
  Top Ten Tunes
  for the Last Fifty Years.
Morrow Quill Paperbacks.
New York, 1981.

Clark, Cynthia &
Chadwick, Donna.
Clinically Adapted
  Instruments for the
  Multiple Handicapped.
Magnamusic-Baton
Music, Inc.
Saint Louis, MO.

Shows how to adapt a variety
of instruments for use by
individuals with various
handicaps. Recommended.

Douglass, Donna.
Accent on Rhythm.
LaRoux Enterprises.
Salem, OR.

Formerly published as
"Happiness is Music!
Music!" "Music!"
Contains "how-to"
information for many
activities.

Drury, Neville.
Music for Inner Space.
Prism Press.

Dylong, John.
Living History, 1925-1950.
Loyola University Press.
Chicago, 1979.

Feil, Naomi.
Validation Therapy.
MMB Music, Inc.
Saint Louis, MO.

Theory and method for
working with the
disoriented elderly.

Gross, Martin A.
Nostalgia Quiz Book
New American Library.
New York, 1969.

Also available as a Signet
paperback

Gutheil, E.
*Music and Your
   Emotions.*
MMB Music, Inc.
Saint Louis, MO

A guide to music selections
with desired emotional
responses.

Halpern, Steve.
*Tuning the Human
   Instrument.*
Halpern Sounds
1775 Old Country Rd., #9
Belmont, CA 94002

Halpern, Steve, and
Savary Louis.
Sound and Health.
Harper and Row, Publishers
New York

Karras, Beckie.
Down Memory Lane.
Circle Press
11821 Idlewood Rd.
Wheaton, MD 20906

Ideas and instruction for
structured reminiscence
groups.

Jones, Bessie, and Hawes,
Bess Lomax.
Step It Down.
Harper and Row, Publishers.
New York, 1972

Games, plays, songs, and
stories from Black
American heritage.

Lingerman, Hal A.
*The Healing Energies
   of Music.*
The Theosophical Publishing
House.

P.O. Box 270.
Wheaton, IL 60187

Miller, Karen J.
Treatment with
  Music: A Manual for
  Allied Health
  Professionals.
Dept. of Occupational
Therapy
College of Health and Human
Services
Western Michigan University
Kalamazoo, MI 49008

Outlines specific techniques
and activities for use with
clients with various
dysfunctions.

Munro, Susan.
Music Therapy in
  Palliative Hospice Care.
MMB Music, Inc.
Saint Louis, MO

Scherman, David, ed.
Life Goes to
  the Movies.
Time/Life Books.
New York, 1975

Scherman, David, ed.
Life Goes to War:
  A Picture History of World
  War II.
Time/Life Books.
New York, 1977

Schwartz, Alvin.
When I Grew Up
  Long Ago.
Lippincott.
New York, 1976

First-person reminiscences.

Sennett, Ted, ed.
Old Time Radio Book.

Pyramid Publications.
New York, 1976

Sennett, Ted, ed.
Hollywood Musicals.
Abrams Publishers.
New York, 1981

Shealy.
The Autoharp.
Lewis Music Publishing Co.
263 Veterans Blvd.
Carlstadt, NJ 07072.

Slabey, Vera.
*Music Involvement
  for Nursing Homes*.
Music Involvement
Mt. Matthew
Durand, WI 54736

A "how-to" book of musical activities.

This Fabulous Century.
Eight volumes:
  V. 1: 1870-1900
  V. 2: 1900-1910
  V. 3: 1910-1920
  V. 4: 1920-1930
  V. 5: 1930-1940
  V. 6: 1940-1950
  V. 7: 1950-1960
  V. 8: 1960-1970
Time/Life Books.
NY, 1969-1970.

An outstanding series which presents detailed information about daily life in each decade. Sadly, out of print. Can sometimes be found in secondhand bookstores. Well worth the time and effort required to find it.

SOURCES FOR RECORDINGS:
NOSTALGIA, MUSICAL ACTIVITIES, GENERAL

Presta Sounds
P.O. Box 368
Cambridge, MA 02141

An excellent source for "nostalgia" music and radio shows, many thematic programs available;

reasonable prices
and excellent service.
Highly recommended.

Recordings for Recovery
Ralph L. Hoy
796 Myers Drive
New Kensington, PA 15068
(412) 339-2422

A free service providing a
variety of music for
therapeutic use. Cassette
tapes available on loan.

Educational Activities, Inc.
Box 392
Freeport, NY 11520

Bowmar Records
10515 Burbank Blvd.
North Hollywood, CA

Teleketics
1229 S. Santee Street
Los Angeles, CA 90015

Folkways Records and Service Corp.
43 W. 61st St.
New York, NY

National Recording
Company
P.O. Box 395
Glenview, IL 60025

Tapes of old radio shows.

SOURCES FOR RECORDINGS:
NEW AGE MUSIC

Rainbow Place
3601 San Mateo Blvd. NE
Albuquerque, NM 87110

Halpern Sounds
1775 Old Country Rd., #9
Belmont, CA 94002

Vital Body Marketing Co.
P.O. Box 703
Fresh Meadows, NY 11365

Source
1307 Buena Vista
Pacific Grove, CA 93950

Backroads
Box 416
Evans, CO 80620

San Francisco Medical Research Foundation
803 Fourth Street
San Rafael, CA 94901

Narada Distributors
1804 E. North Ave.
Milwaukee, WI 53202

Arcana Records
2210 Wilshire Blvd. #348
Santa Monica, CA 90403

Celestial Harmonies
P.O. Box 673
Wilton, CT 06897

Continuum Montage
3107-B Pico Boulevard
Santa Monica, CA 90405

Fortuna Records
P.O. Box 1116
Novato, CA 94947